Procedure Checklists for

Fundamentals of Nursing

HUMAN HEALTH AND FUNCTION

Procedure Checklists for

Fundamentals of Nursing

HUMAN HEALTH AND FUNCTION

SEVENTH EDITION

Ruth F. Craven, EdD, RN, BC, FAAN
Professor Emerita
Department of Behavioral Nursing and Health Systems
University of Washington School of Nursing
Seattle, Washington

Constance J. Hirnle, MN, RN, BC
Clinical Education Specialist
Virginia Mason Medical Center
Seattle, Washington

Senior Lecturer
Biobehavioral Nursing and Health Systems
University of Washington School of Nursing
Seattle, Washington

Sharon Jensen, MN, RN
Instructor
School of Nursing
Seattle University
Seattle, Washington

Wolters Kluwer | Lippincott Williams & Wilkins
Health

Philadelphia • Baltimore • New York • London
Buenos Aires • Hong Kong • Sydney • Tokyo

Executive Acquisitions Editor: Julie Stegman
Senior Product Manager: Michelle Clarke
Senior Designer: Joan Wendt
Manufacturing Coordinator: Karin Duffield
Prepress Vendor: Aptara, Inc.

7th edition

9 8 7 6 5 4 3

Printed in the United States of America.

ISBN: 978-1-60547-787-9

LWW.com

Introduction

Developing clinical competency is an important challenge for each fundamentals nursing student. To facilitate the mastery of nursing skills, we are happy to provide skill checklists for each skill included in *Fundamentals of Nursing: Human Health and Function*, Seventh Edition. Students can use the checklists to facilitate self-evaluation, and faculty will find them useful in measuring and recording student performance. Three-hole-punched and perforated, these checklists can be easily reproduced and brought to the simulation laboratory or clinical area.

The checklists follow each step of the skill to provide a complete evaluative tool. They are designed to record an evaluation of each step of the procedure.

- Checkmark in the "Excellent" column denotes mastering the procedure.
- Checkmark in the "Satisfactory" column indicates use of the recommended technique.
- Checkmark in the "Needs Practice" column indicates use of some but not all of each recommended technique.

The Comments section allows you to highlight suggestions that will improve skills. Space is available at the top of each checklist to record a final pass/fail evaluation, date, and the signature of the student and evaluating faculty member.

List of Procedures by Chapter

Procedure Checklists for

Fundamentals of Nursing

HUMAN HEALTH AND FUNCTION

Procedure Checklist for Fundamentals of Nursing: Human Health and Function, 7th edition

Name ______________________ Date ______________

Unit ______________________ Position ______________

Instructor/Evaluator: ______________________ Position ______________

PROCEDURE 16-1

Measuring Weight

Excellent	Satisfactory	Needs Practice	**Goal:** To provide baseline data from which to assess total fluid balance or nutritional status; to provide baseline data to determine drug dosages or information for diagnostic testing with dye or radioactive injections.	**Comments**
____	____	____	1. Perform hand hygiene.	
____	____	____	2. Identify the patient.	
____	____	____	3. Close door or bed curtains and explain the procedure to the patient.	
____	____	____	4. Have patient void before weighing.	
____	____	____	5. Use the same scale and measure the weight at the same time each day. Patient should wear same clothing for each weight measurement. He or she should remove slippers or shoes before measurement.	
____	____	____	6. Place protective paper or cloth on scale.	
____	____	____	7. Check that scale registers zero. Adjust as necessary.	
			Weight With Standing Scale	
____	____	____	8. Assist patient onto scale. Patient must stand in center of platform and not lean or hold onto supports.	
____	____	____	9. Read digital display or adjust counterweights to determine patient's weight.	
____	____	____	10. Assist patient from scale and record weight in the patient's record.	
			Weight With Chair Scale	
____	____	____	8. Place scale beside patient and lock wheels.	
____	____	____	9. Transfer patient onto chair. If arm of chair is removable, unlock and remove before transfer. Lock back into place after transfer.	
____	____	____	10. Read digital display or adjust counterweights to determine patient's weight.	
____	____	____	11. Transfer patient back to bed or wheelchair.	
____	____	____	12. Clean the scale according to agency policy.	
____	____	____	13. Return scale to proper location and plug in.	

Excellent	Satisfactory	Needs Practice	PROCEDURE 16-1 **Measuring Weight** *(Continued)*	Comments
			Weight With Bed Scale	
____	____	____	8. Elevate patient's bed to level of stretcher scale.	
____	____	____	9. With one or two assistants, turn patient on the side with back toward the scale.	
____	____	____	10. Roll scale toward the bed, lock wheels in place, and lower stretcher onto bed.	
____	____	____	11. Position folded stretcher under patient. Roll patient onto stretcher.	
____	____	____	12. Attach stretcher arms to stretcher and gradually elevate stretcher about 2 inches above mattress surface. Inform patient before elevating. Reassure the patient that he or she will not fall but the head may feel lower than the body.	
____	____	____	13. Determine that the stretcher is not touching any equipment. Lift all drains and tubing away from stretcher.	
____	____	____	14. Read digital display for patient's weight. *Note:* This is a good time to change patient's linen as he or she is elevated off the bed.	
____	____	____	15. Gradually lower stretcher to the bed. Remove stretcher arms and transfer patient off stretcher. Remove stretcher.	
____	____	____	16. Unlock bed scale wheels and move away from bed.	
____	____	____	17. Assist patient to comfortable position.	
____	____	____	18. Clean stretcher and scale according to agency policy. Return to proper location and keep plugged in for next use.	
____	____	____	19. Record weight, and note any extra linen or equipment weighed with the patient.	

Procedure Checklist for Fundamentals of Nursing: Human Health and Function, 7th edition

Name ______________________ Date ______________

Unit ______________________ Position ______________

Instructor/Evaluator: ______________________ Position ______________

PROCEDURE 16-2

Assessing the Neurologic System

Goal: To obtain baseline information about the patient's neurologic status; to assess the patient's orientation to his or her environment; to evaluate the patient's cognitive function and ability to make judgments; to assess the integrity of motor and sensory pathways and the patient's ability to ambulate safely; to detect increased intracranial pressure; to detect changes in neurologic status.

Excellent	Satisfactory	Needs Practice		Comments
____	____	____	1. Perform hand hygiene.	
____	____	____	2. Identify the patient.	
____	____	____	3. Close door or bed curtains and explain the procedure to the patient.	
			Cognitive–Sensory Assessment	
____	____	____	4. Assess the patient's level of consciousness by asking direct questions that require a verbal response. Note appropriateness of response and emotional state.	
____	____	____	5. Evaluate patient's speech patterns.	
____	____	____	6. Observe general appearance: hygiene, appropriateness of clothing to setting and weather.	
____	____	____	7. If patient responses are inappropriate, ask direct questions related to person, place, and time (e.g., "What is your name?" "Where are you right now?" "What city do you live in?" "What day is this?").	
____	____	____	8. If patient doesn't respond or inappropriately responds to orientation questions, give simple commands (e.g., "Squeeze my fingers," "Wiggle your toes"). If the patient gives no response to verbal commands, test response to painful stimuli by applying firm pressure on patient's sternum or fingernail bed with your thumb.	
____	____	____	9. Document cognitive or sensory assessment objectively by stating specific patient responses to verbal or tactile stimulation. Use of Glasgow Coma Scale helps documenting of frequent level-of-consciousness testing.	
____	____	____	10. Assess function of cranial nerves.	

Excellent	Satisfactory	Needs Practice	PROCEDURE 16-2 **Assessing the Neurologic System** *(Continued)*	Comments
___	___	___	11. Assess sensory pathways:	
___	___	___	a. Patient's eyes are closed during all sensory tests.	
___	___	___	b. Apply stimuli to skin in a random, unpredictable order while comparing one side of body with the other.	
___	___	___	c. Patient should verbally state when he or she feels a particular stimulus. If you detect an area of altered sensation, note which spinal cord segment is affected by referring to a dermatome chart.	
___	___	___	12. Test pain sensation first by lightly touching the pointed, then the blunt, end of sterile toothpick to proximal and distal aspects of the arm and legs.	
___	___	___	13. Test temperature sensation by touching skin with vials of hot, then cold, water.	
___	___	___	14. Lightly stroke proximal and distal aspects of patient's arms and legs with a cotton applicator or ball. Ask patient to tell you when and where each stroke is felt.	
___	___	___	15. Apply a vibrating tuning fork to the distal interphalangeal joints of fingers and great toe. Ask patient to describe what he or she feels and when it stops. *Note:* If patient does not feel vibration, move the tuning fork proximally to the next joint until sensation is felt.	
			Activity–Mobility Assessment	
___	___	___	4. Inspect arm and leg muscles for atrophy, tremors, fasciculations, or other abnormal movements.	
___	___	___	5. Assess strength of specific muscle groups by having patient extend or flex individual joints against resistance provided by examiner's hands. Test biceps, triceps, wrist, leg muscles, and ankle.	
___	___	___	6. Ask patient to close eyes and hold arms in front of body with palms up. Have patient hold position for 30 seconds and observe for pronation of hands or drifting of arms (pronator drift). *Note:* Notice weaknesses on one or both sides.	
___	___	___	7. Evaluate coordination and balance.	
___	___	___	a. Perform a series of rapid alternating movements.	
___	___	___	(1) Have patient pat upper thigh by rapidly alternating his or her palm and back of the hand.	

Excellent	Satisfactory	Needs Practice	PROCEDURE 16-2 **Assessing the Neurologic System** *(Continued)*	Comments
___	___	___	(2) With dominant hand, have patient touch his or her thumb to each finger on that hand as quickly as possible.	
___	___	___	(3) Have patient use his or her dominant forefinger to first touch your forefinger, then his or her nose. Instruct patient to repeat this many times as fast as he or she can.	
___	___	___	b. Romberg test: Ask patient to stand with feet together, arms at sides. Have patient maintain this position for 30 seconds with eyes open, then 30 seconds with eyes closed. Assess for swaying. Stay close to patient to assist in case he or she begins to fall.	
___	___	___	c. Ask patient to walk across the room. Observe gait for symmetry, rhythm, limping, shuffling, or other abnormalities.	
___	___	___	8. Assess deep tendon reflexes.	
___	___	___	a. Compare symmetry of reflex on each side of body.	
___	___	___	b. Extremity to be tested should be completely relaxed and slightly extended.	
___	___	___	c. Hold the reflex hammer loosely and allow it to swing freely in an arc.	
___	___	___	d. Tap tendon briskly.	
___	___	___	e. Document reflexes by grading from 0 to 4+ on stick-man, comparing bilaterally.	

Procedure Checklist for Fundamentals of Nursing: Human Health and Function, 7th edition

Name ______________________ Date ______________________

Unit ______________________ Position ______________________

Instructor/Evaluator: ______________________ Position ______________________

PROCEDURE 16-3
Auscultating Breath Sounds

Excellent	Satisfactory	Needs Practice	**Goal**: To listen for variations in breath sounds that may indicate airway obstruction or disease process; to assess the effectiveness of medications or therapies in opening or clearing airways; to detect fluid volume excess or pulmonary edema.	**Comments**
___	___	___	1. Perform hand hygiene.	
___	___	___	2. Identify the patient.	
___	___	___	3. Close door or bed curtains and explain the procedure to the patient.	
___	___	___	4. Assist the patient to an upright sitting position. Remove patient's gown to expose chest.	
___	___	___	5. Warm the diaphragm of the stethoscope by holding it between your hands for a short time.	
___	___	___	6. Ask patient to breathe deeply through the mouth. Patient should breathe slowly.	
			Auscultate Anterior Chest	
___	___	___	7. Place diaphragm of stethoscope about 1 inch below the middle of the right clavicle, making sure it lies between the ribs. Listen to one full inspiration and exhalation. Repeat the process at the corresponding site on the left side.	
___	___	___	8. Note normal and adventitious breath sounds at each point on the chest as you proceed.	
___	___	___	9. Move stethoscope downward about 1.5 to 2 inches along midclavicular line. Note sounds; move stethoscope laterally to opposite side.	
___	___	___	10. Move stethoscope downward another inch or two along midclavicular line to fifth intercostal space. (This space lies just below the nipple line on men, approximately across from the head of the xiphoid process of the sternum.) Note sounds, then move to same spot on opposite side.	
			Auscultate Posterior Chest	
___	___	___	7. Instruct patient to lean forward and cross arms in front.	
___	___	___	8. Begin by auscultating the area about 2 inches below the shoulders and 2 inches to the right of the spine. Note sounds, then move to corresponding point on left.	

PROCEDURE 16-3

Auscultating Breath Sounds *(Continued)*

Excellent	Satisfactory	Needs Practice		Comments
___	___	___	9. Move stethoscope directly downward 2 or 2.5 inches; note sounds, then move stethoscope laterally and listen on the right.	
___	___	___	10. Repeat process, moving downward 2 to 2.5 inches; listen to corresponding opposite side.	
___	___	___	11. Move stethoscope downward to area just below scapula. Listen on right and left. Listen also to areas laterally along lower rib cage.	
___	___	___	12. Replace patient's clothes and assist the patient to a comfortable position.	
___	___	___	13. Discuss your findings with the patient.	
___	___	___	14. Record assessment findings. Be specific as to description and location of adventitious sounds.	

Procedure Checklist for Fundamentals of Nursing: Human Health and Function, 7th edition

Name ______________________________ Date ______________________

Unit ______________________________ Position ______________________

Instructor/Evaluator: ______________________________ Position ______________________

PROCEDURE 16-4
Auscultating Heart Sounds

Goal: To assess normal and abnormal functioning of the heart valves; to detect cardiac problems.

Excellent	Satisfactory	Needs Practice		Comments
____	____	____	1. Perform hand hygiene.	
____	____	____	2. Identify the patient.	
____	____	____	3. Close door or bed curtains and explain the procedure to the patient.	
____	____	____	4. Assist the patient to the supine position for auscultation. You may want to re-examine the patient in the upright sitting position and a left lateral position. Lift patient's gown to expose the chest.	
____	____	____	5. Warm the diaphragm of the stethoscope by holding it between your hands for a few moments.	
____	____	____	6. Listen in the mitral area using the diaphragm. Identify the first and second heart sounds (S_1 and S_2). Count the heart rate, noting whether the rhythm is regular or irregular. If the rhythm is irregular, count the heart rate for a full minute. Also note whether the irregularity has a pattern or whether it is totally unpredictable.	
____	____	____	7. Listen in the aortic area using the diaphragm. Concentrate first on S_1, then S_2, noting whether splitting occurs. Shift your concentration to systole and then diastole; listen for extra sounds, such as murmurs.	
____	____	____	8. Listen in the pulmonic area, still using only the diaphragm. Repeat the sequence described in step 5, concentrating on S_1, S_2, systole, and diastole. Compare the loudness of S_2 in the aortic and pulmonic areas.	
____	____	____	9. Move the diaphragm and listen to the tricuspid and mitral areas.	
____	____	____	10. Return to the aortic area, this time using the bell of the stethoscope. As before, concentrate individually on S_1, S_2, systole, and diastole.	
____	____	____	11. Repeat the same process, using the bell, in the pulmonic, tricuspid, and mitral areas. Especially in the mitral area, concentrate during diastole to detect a third or fourth heart sound (S_3 and S_4).	
____	____	____	12. Replace the patient's clothes. Assist the patient to a comfortable position.	
____	____	____	13. Record your assessment findings, describing the intensity, quality, and location of the sounds.	

Procedure Checklist for Fundamentals of Nursing: Human Health and Function, 7th edition

Name ______________________ Date ______________________

Unit ______________________ Position ______________________

Instructor/Evaluator: ______________________ Position ______________________

PROCEDURE 16-5
Auscultating Bowel Sounds

Excellent	Satisfactory	Needs Practice	**Goal:** To determine the presence or absence of intestinal peristalsis.	Comments
____	____	____	1. Perform hand hygiene.	
____	____	____	2. Identify the patient.	
____	____	____	3. Close door or bed curtains and explain the procedure to the patient.	
____	____	____	4. Ask the patient when he or she last ate.	
____	____	____	5. Have the patient urinate before the examination.	
____	____	____	6. Assist the patient to a supine position with abdomen exposed.	
____	____	____	7. Visually divide the abdomen into four quadrants using the umbilicus as the central crossing landmark.	
____	____	____	8. Place the stethoscope diaphragm in each of the four quadrants. Listen for pitch, frequency, and duration of bowel sounds at each site.	
____	____	____	9. If you do not hear bowel sounds, listen for 3 to 5 minutes in all quadrants before concluding that they are absent.	
____	____	____	10. Proceed with the rest of the physical examination or cover the patient's abdomen and assist him or her to a comfortable position.	
____	____	____	11. Document your findings.	

Procedure Checklist for Fundamentals of Nursing: Human Health and Function, 7th edition

Name ______________________ Date ______________________

Unit ______________________ Position ______________________

Instructor/Evaluator: ______________________ Position ______________________

PROCEDURE 17-1

Assessing Body Temperature

Excellent	Satisfactory	Needs Practice	**Goal:** Obtain baseline temperature data for comparing future measurements; screen for alterations in temperature; evaluate temperature response to therapies.	Comments
___	___	___	1. Perform hand hygiene.	
___	___	___	2. Identify the patient.	
___	___	___	3. Close door or bed curtains, and explain the procedure to the patient.	
			Assessing Oral Temperature With an Electronic Thermometer	
___	___	___	4. Remove electronic thermometer from the battery pack, and remove the temperature probe from the recording unit, noting a digital display of temperature on the screen (usually 34°C [94°F]).	
___	___	___	5. Place the disposable cover over the temperature probe and attach securely. Grasp the base of the probe.	
___	___	___	6. Insert the probe below the patient's tongue and into the posterior sublingual pocket of the mouth. Ask the patient to close his or her lips around the probe. Hold the probe, supporting it in place.	
___	___	___	7. Wait for a beep (usually 10 to 20 seconds), which indicates the estimated temperature. Watch to see if temperature continues to rise. When the temperature reading stops rising, note the temperature displayed on the unit and remove the probe from the patient's mouth.	
___	___	___	8. Hold the probe over a waste container, and displace the probe cover by pressing the probe release button.	
___	___	___	9. Return the probe to the storage place within the unit, and return the thermometer to the battery pack. Cleanse according to agency policy.	
___	___	___	10. Record temperature on vital sign documentation record, indicating "O" for oral site. Discuss findings with patient if appropriate.	
			Assessing Rectal Temperature With an Electronic Thermometer	
___	___	___	4. Assist patient to Sims' position with upper leg flexed. Expose only anal area.	

Excellent	Satisfactory	Needs Practice	PROCEDURE 17-1 **Assessing Body Temperature** *(Continued)*	Comments
____	____	____	5. Remove rectal (red) electronic thermometer from battery pack, and extend the temperature probe from the unit, noting a digital display of temperature on the screen.	
____	____	____	6. Securely attach the disposable cover over the temperature probe.	
____	____	____	7. Apply water-soluble lubricant liberally to thermometer probe tip.	
____	____	____	8. Separate patient's buttocks with one gloved hand until the anal sphincter is visible.	
____	____	____	9. Ask patient to take a deep, slow breath. Insert thermometer into anus in direction of umbilicus, 1 inch (2.5 cm) for a child and 1.5 inches (4 cm) for an adult. Do not force.	
____	____	____	10. Hold the probe in place until machine emits a beep. Obtain reading.	
____	____	____	11. Follow steps 7 through 9 in Assessing Oral Temperature With an Electronic Thermometer. Document "R" for rectal site.	
			Assessing Temperature Using a Tympanic Membrane Thermometer	
____	____	____	4. Remove tympanic thermometer from recharging base, and check that the lens is clean. Attach tympanic probe cover to sensor unit.	
____	____	____	5. Insert probe into ear canal, making sure the probe fits snugly. Avoid forcing the probe too deeply into the ear. Pulling the pinna back, up, and out in an adult will straighten the ear canal. Some manufacturers recommend moving the thermometer in a figure eight pattern. Rotate the probe handle toward the jawline.	
____	____	____	6. Activate the thermometer, and note the temperature readout, which is usually displayed within 2 seconds.	
____	____	____	7. Eject sensor probe cover directly into waste container, cleanse according to agency policy, and return tympanic thermometer to base for storage or recharging. Store away from temperature extremes.	
____	____	____	8. Record temperature on vital sign documentation record. Document "TM" for tympanic membrane site. Discuss findings with patient if appropriate.	
			Assessing Temperature Using a Temporal Artery Thermometer	
____	____	____	4. Remove thermometer from storage base. If low battery indicator shows, replace battery.	

Excellent	Satisfactory	Needs Practice	PROCEDURE 17-1 **Assessing Body Temperature** *(Continued)*	Comments
___	___	___	5. Inspect the thermometer lens. If not shiny, clean by first wiping with alcohol, then rinsing with water-dampened swabs. Allow to air dry. Lens should be cleaned daily.	
___	___	___	6. Attach disposable cover.	
___	___	___	7. Move hair to expose forehead and hairline. Measure only exposed side of forehead. If patient is lying on side, measure "up" side only. If patient is perspiring heavily (diaphoretic), consider alternate method (e.g., oral).	
___	___	___	8. Place probe flush against the center of the forehead and depress button. Slowly slide probe straight across forehead to hairline. Keeping button depressed, lift the probe from the forehead and touch it briefly against the neck just behind the earlobe.	
___	___	___	9. Release the button and read the recorded temperature within 15 seconds. If repeated measurements are necessary, wait at least 30 seconds.	
___	___	___	10. Eject probe cover directly into waste container or keep at bedside to use again on the same patient, cleanse according to agency policy, and return temporal thermometer to storage base. Store away from temperature extremes.	
___	___	___	11. Record temperature on vital sign documentation record, indicating "TA" for temporal artery site. Discuss findings with patient if appropriate.	
			Assessing Axillary Temperature With an Electronic Thermometer	
___	___	___	7. Assist patient to comfortable position, and remove clothing to expose axilla.	
___	___	___	8. Place thermometer against middle of axilla; fold patient's arm down and place across chest, enclosing thermometer in axillary area.	
___	___	___	9. Wait for a beep that indicates the estimated temperature. Watch to see if temperature continues to rise. When it stops, note the temperature displayed on the unit and remove the probe from the patient's axilla.	
___	___	___	10. Follow steps 8 and 9 in Assessing Oral Temperature With an Electronic Thermometer. Document "A" for axillary site.	

Procedure Checklist for Fundamentals of Nursing: Human Health and Function, 7th edition

Name ______________________ Date ______________

Unit ______________________ Position ______________

Instructor/Evaluator: ______________________ Position ______________

PROCEDURE 17-2

Obtaining a Pulse

Excellent	Satisfactory	Needs Practice	**Goal:** Obtain a baseline measurement of heart rate and rhythm; evaluate the heart's response to various therapies and medications; peripheral pulse may be palpated to assess local blood flow to an extremity or to monitor perfusion to an extremity following surgery or diagnostic procedures (e.g., cardiac catheterization).	Comments
____	____	____	1. Perform hand hygiene.	
____	____	____	2. Identify the patient.	
____	____	____	3. Close door or bed curtains and explain the procedure to the patient.	
			Obtaining a Radial Pulse	
____	____	____	4. Position patient comfortably with forearm across chest or at side with wrist extended.	
____	____	____	5. Place fingertips of your first two or three fingers along the groove at base of thumb, on patient's wrist.	
____	____	____	6. Press against radial artery to obliterate pulse, then gradually release pressure until you feel pulsations; assess for regularity and strength.	
____	____	____	7. If pulse is not easily palpable, use Doppler.	
____	____	____	a. Apply conducting gel to end of probe or to radial site.	
____	____	____	b. Press "on" button and place probe against skin on pulse site. Reposition slightly, using firm pressure, until you hear a pulsating sound.	
____	____	____	8. If pulse is regular, count pulse for 30 seconds and then multiply by two. If pulse is irregular, count for 1 full minute. If irregular pulse is a new finding, assess apical-radial rate. Count the initial pulse as zero.	
			Obtaining an Apical Pulse	
____	____	____	4. Position patient in supine or sitting position with sternum and left chest exposed.	
____	____	____	5. Warm diaphragm of stethoscope by holding it in the palm of your hand for 5 to 10 seconds.	
____	____	____	6. Use an alcohol swab to clean the stethoscope and earpieces before using.	

PROCEDURE 17-2

Obtaining a Pulse *(Continued)*

Excellent	Satisfactory	Needs Practice		Comments
____	____	____	7. Locate apex of the patient's heart by palpating the space between the fifth and sixth rib (fifth intercostal space) and moving to the left midclavicular line.	
____	____	____	8. Insert the earpieces of stethoscope into your ears, and place diaphragm over apex of patient's heart.	
____	____	____	9. Assess the heartbeat for regularity and dysrhythmias.	
____	____	____	10. If rhythm is regular, count the heartbeat for 30 seconds and then multiply by two. Count for 1 full minute if the rhythm is irregular. Count the initial pulse as zero.	
____	____	____	11. Replace the patient's gown and assist the patient to return to a comfortable position.	
____	____	____	12. Share results of assessment with patient, if appropriate.	
____	____	____	13. Document pulse on vital sign record or computerized record. Specify in the documentation that you obtained an apical pulse (e.g., "AP").	

Procedure Checklist for Fundamentals of Nursing: Human Health and Function, 7th edition

Name ______________________ Date ______________________

Unit ______________________ Position ______________________

Instructor/Evaluator: ______________________ Position ______________________

PROCEDURE 17-3

Assessing Respirations

Goal: Assess respiratory status by evaluating rate and quality; evaluate the influence of medications and therapies on respiration.

Excellent	Satisfactory	Needs Practice	Step	Comments
___	___	___	1. Perform hand hygiene.	
___	___	___	2. Identify the patient.	
___	___	___	3. Close door or bed curtains and explain the procedure to the patient.	
___	___	___	4. After or before assessment of pulse, keep your fingers resting on patient's wrist and observe or feel the rising and falling of chest with respiration. If patient is asleep, you may gently place your hand on the patient's chest so you can feel chest movement. Do not explain procedure to patient.	
___	___	___	5. When you have observed one complete cycle of inspiration and expiration, and if respiration is regular, look at second hand of your watch and count the number of complete cycles in 1 full minute.	
___	___	___	6. If respirations are shallow and difficult to count, observe at the sternal notch.	
___	___	___	7. Note depth and rhythm of respiratory cycle.	
___	___	___	8. Discuss findings with patient and document respiratory rate, depth, rhythm, and character.	

Procedure Checklist for Fundamentals of Nursing: Human Health and Function, 7th edition

Name ______________________ Date ______________

Unit ______________________ Position ______________

Instructor/Evaluator: ______________________ Position ______________

PROCEDURE 17-4

Obtaining Blood Pressure

Goal: Evaluate the patient's hemodynamic status by obtaining information about cardiac output, blood volume, peripheral vascular resistance, and arterial wall elasticity; obtain baseline measurement of blood pressure; monitor the hemodynamic response to various therapies or disease conditions; screen for hypertension.

Excellent	Satisfactory	Needs Practice	Step	Comments
___	___	___	1. Perform hand hygiene.	
___	___	___	2. Identify the patient.	
___	___	___	3. Close door or bed curtains and explain the procedure to the patient.	
___	___	___	4. Clean stethoscope head with alcohol or approved cleaning solution.	
___	___	___	5. Assist patient to a comfortable position with forearm supported at heart level and palm up. Verify that you have a correctly sized blood pressure cuff.	
___	___	___	6. Expose the upper arm completely. Palpate the brachial artery.	
___	___	___	7. Wrap deflated cuff snugly around upper arm with center of bladder over brachial artery. Lower border of cuff should be about 2 cm above the antecubital space (nearer the antecubital space on an infant).	
___	___	___	8. Palpate brachial or radial artery with fingertips. Close valve on pressure bulb and inflate cuff until pulse disappears. Slowly release valve and note reading when pulse reappears.	
___	___	___	9. Fully deflate cuff and wait 1 to 2 minutes.	
___	___	___	10. Place stethoscope earpiece in ears. Repalpate the brachial artery, and place stethoscope bell or diaphragm over site.	
___	___	___	11. Close bulb valve by turning clockwise. Ensure gauge starts at zero. Pump bulb to inflate cuff. Inflate cuff to 30 mm Hg above reading where brachial pulse disappeared.	
___	___	___	12. Open valve on manometer, then slowly release valve so pressure drops about 2 to 3 mm Hg per second.	
___	___	___	13. Identify manometer reading when first clear Korotkoff sound is heard.	
___	___	___	14. Continue to deflate, and note reading when sound muffles or dampens (fourth Korotkoff) and when it disappears (fifth Korotkoff).	

Excellent	Satisfactory	Needs Practice	PROCEDURE 17-4 **Obtaining Blood Pressure** *(Continued)*	Comments
____	____	____	15. Deflate cuff completely and remove from patient's arm.	
____	____	____	16. If cuff will be used on another patient, clean cuff according to agency requirements and allow to air-dry.	
____	____	____	17. Record blood pressure. Record systolic (e.g., 130) and diastolic (e.g., 80) in the form "130/80." If three pressures are to be recorded, use the form "130/80/40" (40 is the fifth Korotkoff). Abbreviate as "RA" or "LA" to indicate right or left arm measurement.	
____	____	____	18. Assist patient to comfortable position and discuss findings with patient, if appropriate.	

Procedure Checklist for Fundamentals of Nursing: Human Health and Function, 7th edition

Name ______________________ Date ______________________

Unit ______________________ Position ______________________

Instructor/Evaluator: ______________________ Position ______________________

PROCEDURE 17-5

Assessing for Orthostatic Hypotension

Goal: Assess the compensatory status of the cardiovascular and autonomic nervous systems to changes in body position; assess for fluid volume deficit; assess patient's safety in getting up and ambulating.

Excellent	Satisfactory	Needs Practice	Steps	Comments
___	___	___	1. Perform hand hygiene.	
___	___	___	2. Identify the patient.	
___	___	___	3. Close door or bed curtains and explain the procedure to the patient.	
___	___	___	4. Position patient supine with head of bed flat for 10 minutes.	
___	___	___	5. Check and record supine blood pressure and pulse. Keep blood pressure cuff attached.	
___	___	___	6. Assist patient to a sitting position at edge of bed with feel flat on the floor. Wait 2 to 4 minutes and check blood pressure and pulse rate. *Note:* The waiting period is a convenient time to auscultate the patient's lung fields.	
___	___	___	7. Assist patient to standing position, then wait 2 to 4 minutes and check blood pressure and pulse rate. Be alert to signs and symptoms of dizziness.	
___	___	___	8. Assist the patient back to a comfortable position.	
___	___	___	9. Record measurements and any symptoms that accompanied the postural change. Report a drop of 25 mm Hg in systolic pressure or a drop of 10 mm Hg in diastolic pressure.	
___	___	___	10. Discuss findings with patient, if appropriate.	

Procedure Checklist for Fundamentals of Nursing: Human Health and Function, 7th edition

Name ______________________________ Date ______________

Unit ______________________________ Position ______________

Instructor/Evaluator: ______________________ Position ______________

PROCEDURE 18-1

Hand Hygiene

Goal: Reduce the numbers of resident and transient bacteria on the hands; prevent transfer of microorganisms from healthcare personnel to the patient.

Excellent	Satisfactory	Needs Practice	Step	Comments
___	___	___	1. Remove all rings except a plain wedding band. Push watch 4 to 5 inches above wrist.	
___	___	___	2. Turn on the water and adjust temperature to warm. Do not splash water or lean against the wet sink. Faucets may be controlled by your hands or may be operated by knee levers or foot pedals.	
___	___	___	3. Hold hands lower than elbows and thoroughly wet hands and lower arms under running water.	
___	___	___	4. Apply soap and rub palms, wrists, and back of hands firmly with circular movements. Interlace fingers and thumbs, moving hands back and forth. Wash at least 1 inch above the area of contamination. If there is no visible soiling, wash to 1 inch above wrists. Continue using plenty of lather and friction for 15 to 30 seconds on each hand. Timing of scrub may vary depending on purpose of wash and amount of contamination.	
___	___	___	5. Clean under fingernails using fingernails of other hand and additional soap. Use orangewood stick if available.	
___	___	___	6. Rinse hands and wrists thoroughly with hands held lower than forearms.	
___	___	___	7. Dry hands and arms thoroughly with paper towel, wiping from fingertips toward forearm. Discard paper towel in proper receptacle.	
___	___	___	8. Turn off water using clean, dry paper towel on faucets.	
___	___	___	9. Apply oil-free lotion, especially if skin is dry.	

Procedure Checklist for Fundamentals of Nursing: Human Health and Function, 7th edition

Name ______________________ Date ______________________

Unit ______________________ Position ______________________

Instructor/Evaluator: ______________________ Position ______________________

PROCEDURE 18-2

Applying and Removing Personal Protective Equipment

Excellent	Satisfactory	Needs Practice	**Goal:** Prevent transfer of microorganisms via the contact, droplet, and airborne modes of transmission from one patient to another; prevent transmission of microorganisms to self or clothing during patient care.	**Comments**
___	___	___	1. Perform hand hygiene.	
			Applying PPE	
___	___	___	2. Unfold the gown in front of you.	
___	___	___	3. Place your arms through the sleeves and tie at the neck and back.	
___	___	___	4. Place the mask at your lower face, secure around ears, and pull down the mask to cover below chin and fit the nose area securely. If the mask has ties, secure the ties above the ears and around the neck. When wearing glasses, be sure to position the mask edge under the glasses. Make sure the mask fits securely and comfortably.	
___	___	___	5. If splash is anticipated, put on goggles or face shield, making sure they fit securely. Alternatively, a face shield with mask can take the place of the mask and goggles.	
___	___	___	6. Don gloves last so that the cuffs of the gloves fit snugly over the cuffs of the gown.	
			Removing PPE	
___	___	___	1. Remain inside the patient's door while removing PPE. PPE must never be reused.	
___	___	___	2. To remove gloves: First slide your thumb under the cuff of the glove and pull it inside out off your hand. Continue to hold the discarded glove in the other gloved hand and perform the same removal procedure, turning the glove inside out over the discarded glove. Dispose in appropriate waste container. Wash hands.	
___	___	___	3. To remove goggles or face shield: Hold only the headband or ear pieces. Lift away from the face. Place in designated receptacle for reprocessing or in an appropriate waste container.	

PROCEDURE 18-2

Applying and Removing Personal Protective Equipment *(Continued)*

Excellent	Satisfactory	Needs Practice		Comments
____	____	____	4. To remove gown: Untie and pull the gown away from you near the neck, grasping from the inside and avoiding touching the outside. Roll it into a ball, inside out, and keep the sleeves inside the ball. Discard in appropriate waste container.	
____	____	____	5. To remove mask: Hold only by earbands or ties (bottom tie first, then top) and move the mask away from the face. Discard in appropriate waste container.	
____	____	____	6. Wash hands thoroughly with an alcohol-based hand sanitizer unless hands are visibly soiled; if they are, use soap and warm water. If the patient has diarrhea or the Norovirus, use soap and water.	

Procedure Checklist for Fundamentals of Nursing: Human Health and Function, 7th edition

Name ______________________ Date ______________________

Unit ______________________ Position ______________________

Instructor/Evaluator: ______________________ Position ______________________

PROCEDURE 18-3

Preparing and Maintaining a Sterile Field

Excellent	Satisfactory	Needs Practice	**Goal**: Create an environment to prevent the transfer of microorganisms during sterile procedures; create an environment that helps ensure the sterility of supplies and equipment during a sterile procedure.	Comments
			Preparing a Sterile Field Using a Commercially Prepared Sterile Kit or Tray	
____	____	____	1. Perform hand hygiene.	
____	____	____	2. Inspect the sterile kit for package integrity, contamination, or moisture.	
____	____	____	3. During the entire procedure, never turn your back on the sterile field or lower your hands below the level of the field.	
____	____	____	4. Remove the sterile drape from the outer wrapper and place the inner drape in the center of the work surface, at or above waist level, with the outer flap facing away from you.	
____	____	____	5. Touching the outside of the flap only, reach around (rather than over) the sterile field to open the flap away from you.	
____	____	____	6. Open the side flaps in the same manner, using the right hand for the right flap and the left hand for the left flap.	
____	____	____	7. Last, open the innermost flap that faces you, being careful that it does not touch your clothing or any object.	
			Preparing a Sterile Field Using a Packaged Sterile Drape	
____	____	____	1. Open the outer covering of the drape.	
____	____	____	2. Remove the sterile drape by carefully pinching over the top edge (1 inch) of the two corners so that you are touching only the underneath of the sterile drape (bottom, moisture-proof side). Lift the drape carefully out of the package, holding it away from your body and above your waist and work surface.	
____	____	____	3. Continuing to hold only by the pinched-over corners, allow the drape to unfold away from your body and any other surface.	
____	____	____	4. Position the drape on the work surface with the moisture-proof side down (shiny or blue side). Avoid touching any other surface or object with the drape.	

Excellent	Satisfactory	Needs Practice	PROCEDURE 18-3 **Preparing and Maintaining a Sterile Field** *(Continued)*	Comments
			Adding Sterile Supplies to the Field	
___	___	___	5. Open prepackaged sterile supplies by peeling back the partially sealed edge with both hands or lifting up the unsealed edge, taking care not to touch the supplies with your hands.	
___	___	___	6. Hold supplies 6 to 8 inches above the field and allow them to fall to the middle of the sterile field.	
___	___	___	7. Add wrapped sterile supplies by grasping the sterile object with one hand and unwrapping the flaps with the other hand.	
___	___	___	8. Grasp the corners of the wrapper with the free hand and hold them against the wrist of the other hand while you carefully drop the object onto the middle of the sterile field.	
			Adding Solutions to a Sterile Field	
___	___	___	9. Read the solution label and expiration date. Note any signs of contamination.	
___	___	___	10. Remove cap and place it with the inside facing up on a flat surface. Do not touch inside of cap or rim of bottle.	
___	___	___	11. If bottle has been opened previously, "lip" it by pouring a small amount of solution into a waste container.	
___	___	___	12. Hold the bottle 6 inches above container on the sterile field and pour slowly to avoid spills. Label solution.	
___	___	___	13. Recap the solution bottle and label it with date and time of opening if the solution is to be reused.	
___	___	___	14. Add any additional supplies and don sterile gloves before starting the procedure.	

Procedure Checklist for Fundamentals of Nursing: Human Health and Function, 7th edition

Name ______________________ Date ______________

Unit ______________________ Position ______________

Instructor/Evaluator: ______________________ Position ______________

PROCEDURE 18-4

Applying and Removing Sterile Gloves

Excellent	Satisfactory	Needs Practice	**Goal**: Prevent transfer of microorganisms from hands to sterile objects or open wounds.	Comments
			Applying Gloves	
___	___	___	1. Perform hand hygiene.	
___	___	___	2. Remove outside wrapper by peeling apart sides.	
___	___	___	3. Lay inner package on clean, flat surface about waist level. Open wrapper from the outside, keeping gloves on inside surface.	
___	___	___	4. Grasp inside edge of the folded cuff of glove with thumb and first two fingers of your dominant hand. Holding hands above waist, insert your nondominant hand into glove. Leave the cuff folded until the opposite hand is gloved.	
___	___	___	5. Slip gloved hand inside the second gloved cuff still in package and pull over dominant hand, extending the cuff down the arm. Hold gloved thumb out of the way so it doesn't come in contact with ungloved hand.	
___	___	___	6. Keeping hands above waist, adjust fingers inside the glove, touching only sterile areas.	
			Removing Gloves	
___	___	___	7. With dominant hand, grasp outer surface of nondominant glove just below thumb. Peel off without touching exposed wrist.	
___	___	___	8. Place ungloved hand under thumb side of second cuff and peel off toward the fingers, holding first glove inside second glove. Discard into appropriate receptacle.	
___	___	___	9. Complete hand hygiene.	

Procedure Checklist for Fundamentals of Nursing: Human Health and Function, 7th edition

Name ____________________ Date ____________________

Unit ____________________ Position ____________________

Instructor/Evaluator: ____________________ Position ____________________

PROCEDURE 19-1

Administering Oral Medications

Excellent	Satisfactory	Needs Practice	**Goal**: Provide a safe, effective, economical route for administering medications; provide sustained drug action with minimal discomfort	**Comments**
___	___	___	1. Review physician's orders for accuracy and completeness, including patient's name, drug name, dosage, route, and time and indications.	
___	___	___	2. Perform hand hygiene.	
___	___	___	3. Arrange MAR next to medication supply.	
___	___	___	4. Prepare medications for only one patient at a time. Check patient allergies before removing any medications.	
___	___	___	5. Remove ordered medications from supply. Compare label on medication with the MAR or EMAR, and check the six rights of medication administration. Scan bar code if using BCMA. If a discrepancy exists, recheck the patient's chart and medication orders.	
___	___	___	6. Calculate correct drug dosage if necessary.	
___	___	___	7. Prepare selected medications.	
___	___	___	a. Unit dosage: Place packaged medications directly into medicine cup or lay them on tray without unwrapping them.	
___	___	___	b. Medications from a multidose bottle: Pour tablets or capsules into the container lid, and transfer them into medicine cup. Return any extra tablets to the bottle. Label all unlabeled medications. Break only scored tablets, if necessary, using a pill cutter to obtain proper dosage.	
___	___	___	c. Medications from a bingo card: Snap the bubble containing the correct medication directly over the medication cup. Do not touch the medication.	
___	___	___	d. Swallowing difficulty: If patient has trouble swallowing tablets, grind with mortar and pestle or other drug-crushing device until smooth. Mix powder in small amount of pudding or applesauce. Do not crush enteric-coated tablets or extended-release tablets.	

PROCEDURE 19-1

Administering Oral Medications *(Continued)*

Excellent	Satisfactory	Needs Practice		Comments
___	___	___	e. Liquid medications: Remove cap and place on countertop with the inside up. Hold bottle so label is against palm of hand. Fill until bottom of meniscus (the surface of the fluid that appears curved) is at desired dosage. Discard excess poured liquid from cup into sink; do not pour it back into the bottle. Label medication.	
___	___	___	8. Take medications directly to patient's room. Keep medications in sight at all times.	
___	___	___	9. Compare name on MAR with name on patient's identification band using two separate identifiers (e.g., name, MRN, Social Security number, or birth date). Do not administer medications if the patient is not wearing an identification band. Scan patient's identification bracelet if using BCMA.	
___	___	___	10. Complete any preadministration assessment (e.g., blood pressure, pulse) required for the specific medication to be given.	
___	___	___	11. Compare medication to MAR, and recheck the six rights of medication administration. If using unit-dose medication, unwrap the medication and place it in the cup before checking the six rights of the next medication.	
___	___	___	12. Explain the medication's purpose to the patient.	
___	___	___	13. Assist patient to sitting position if necessary. Give the medication cup and glass of water to the patient.	
___	___	___	14. If patient cannot hold the medication cup, place it to the patient's lips and introduce the medication into his or her mouth. If a tablet or capsule falls on the floor, discard and repeat preparation.	
___	___	___	15. Stay with patient until he or she swallows all medications. Look inside patient's mouth if the patient is cognitively impaired or has difficulty swallowing.	
___	___	___	16. Dispose of soiled supplies, and wash hands.	
___	___	___	17. Document time at which medication was administered and any preadministration assessment in order data collected. Note the time that postadministration assessments to assess effectiveness are due for prn medications. If a medication has been held, note this (usually by circling initials on the MAR in the applicable time slot) and give the reason the medication was not given.	

Procedure Checklist for Fundamentals of Nursing: Human Health and Function, 7th edition

Name ______________________ Date ______________________

Unit ______________________ Position ______________________

Instructor/Evaluator: ______________________ Position ______________________

PROCEDURE 19-2

Administering Medication by Metered-Dose Inhaler

Excellent	Satisfactory	Needs Practice	**Goal:** Deliver a premeasured dose of medication to the bronchial airways and lungs	Comments
____	____	____	1. Review physician's order for type of medication, dosage, and route, and assess patient allergies (see Procedure 19-1, steps 1 through 6).	
____	____	____	2. Identify the patient.	
____	____	____	3. Close door or bed curtains and explain the procedure to the patient.	
____	____	____	4. Assist the patient to sitting or standing position. Perform the second medication check of six rights.	
____	____	____	5. Instruct the patient on assembly of medication canister, inhalation mouthpiece, and spacer device if needed. Instruct the patient to attach the medication canister to the inhaler mouthpiece by inserting the metal stem into the long end of the mouthpiece. Teach patient to shake the canister and spacer several times.	
____	____	____	6. Steps 6 through 8 need to occur smoothly, one right after the other. Ask patient to breathe out through his or her mouth.	
____	____	____	7. Assist the patient to position the mouthpiece 1 to 2 inches from his or her open mouth. If using a spacer, have patient place spacer's mouthpiece into mouth, forming a secure seal. Instruct the patient to breathe in slowly through the mouth. As the patient starts inhaling, instruct the patient to press the canister down to release one dose of the medication.	
____	____	____	8. Instruct the patient to hold his or her breath for 10 seconds (if possible) and then to exhale slowly through pursed lips.	
____	____	____	9. Wait at least 1 minute before administration of a second puff by MDI.	
____	____	____	10. Wash hands and clean mouthpiece. If steroid medication was administered, have patient rinse mouth.	
____	____	____	11. Reassess ease of breathing, respiratory rate, accessory muscle use, and breath sounds.	

Excellent	Satisfactory	Needs Practice	PROCEDURE 19-2 **Administering Medication by Metered-Dose Inhaler** *(Continued)*	Comments
____	____	____	12. Document medication administration and patient status before and after administration.	
			Modification for Using a Spacer With a Metered-Dose Inhaler	
____	____	____	13. Attach the spacer to the inhaler mouthpiece. Instruct the patient to exhale and then place the mouthpiece in the mouth, closing his or her lips around the mouthpiece. Depress the medication canister and have the patient inhale until the medication from the chamber is gone. Advise the patient to take two or three short breaths to get all the medication from the spacer.	

Procedure Checklist for Fundamentals of Nursing: Human Health and Function, 7th edition

Name ______________________ Date ______________________

Unit ______________________ Position ______________________

Instructor/Evaluator: ______________________ Position ______________________

PROCEDURE 19-3

Withdrawing Medication From a Vial

Excellent	Satisfactory	Needs Practice	**Goal:** Withdraw a precise amount of medication from a vial while maintaining asepsis.	**Comments**
____	____	____	1. Check medication order and compare the name of the ordered medication with the label on the medication vial. Complete steps 1 through 6 in Procedure 19-1.	
____	____	____	2. Assemble needle and syringe.	
____	____	____	3. Pick up vial. If medication has been reconstituted or is in suspension, place the vial between your palms, rotating or rolling the vial back and forth. Do not shake the vial.	
____	____	____	4. Remove metal cap from vial, cleanse top of vial with alcohol wipe, and remove guard from needle. If multidose vial is being used (e.g., withdrawing insulin), date the vial when opened and discard on expiration date. Cleanse the vial top with alcohol prior to withdrawal.	
____	____	____	5. Pull back on barrel of syringe to draw in a volume of air equal to the volume of the ordered medication dose. Holding the vial between the thumb and fingers of the nondominant hand, insert needle through the rubber stopper into the air space—not the solution—in the vial and inject air.	
____	____	____	6. Invert the vial and withdraw the ordered dose of medication by pulling back on the plunger. Make sure that the needle is in the solution to be withdrawn (look at vial for fluid versus air).	
____	____	____	7. Expel air bubbles and adjust dose if necessary.	
____	____	____	8. Remove needle from vial and cover the needle with guard. Perform hand hygiene.	

Procedure Checklist for Fundamentals of Nursing: Human Health and Function, 7th edition

Name ______________________ Date ______________________

Unit ______________________ Position ______________________

Instructor/Evaluator: ______________________ Position ______________________

PROCEDURE 19-4

Withdrawing Medication From an Ampule

Excellent	Satisfactory	Needs Practice	**Goal:** Withdraw the full dose of medication from an ampule safely while maintaining asepsis.	Comments
____	____	____	1. Check medication order and make sure the solution in the ampule matches the ordered solution. Complete steps 1 through 6 in Procedure 19-1.	
____	____	____	2. Assemble filter needle and syringe.	
____	____	____	3. Pick up ampule and flick its upper stem several times with a fingernail.	
____	____	____	4. Wrap a sterile gauze pad or alcohol wipe around the ampule's neck before breaking the neck along the scored line with an outward snapping motion. Always break away from your body.	
____	____	____	5. Discard the broken neck appropriately, and prepare to withdraw medication from the ampule using one of the following methods:	
____	____	____	a. Place the ampule upright on a flat surface, insert the needle in the solution, and withdraw the correct amount of medication by pulling up on the plunger. Do not touch the needle to the glass rim.	
____	____	____	b. Tilt the ampule sideways. Withdraw the proper dose of medication.	
____	____	____	6. Remove the needle from the solution. Hold the needle upright, inspect the syringe, and dispel any air that may have been drawn into the syringe. Make sure that the syringe contains the right amount of medication. Expel any extra medication. Label syringe.	
____	____	____	7. Cover the filter needle with a safety guard and change the needle. Discard ampule in sharps container.	
____	____	____	8. Perform hand hygiene.	

Procedure Checklist for Fundamentals of Nursing: Human Health and Function, 7th edition

Name ______________________ Date ______________________

Unit ______________________ Position ______________________

Instructor/Evaluator: ______________________ Position ______________________

PROCEDURE 19-5

Drawing Up Two Medications in a Syringe

Excellent	Satisfactory	Needs Practice	**Goal:** Minimize the number of injections a patient receives; prevent contaminating one vial of medication with medication from the other vial.	**Comments**
___	___	___	1. Check medication order and compare the name of the ordered medication with the label on the medication vial. Complete steps 1 through 6 in Procedure 19-1.	
___	___	___	2. Cleanse tops of both vials with antiseptic.	
___	___	___	3. With syringe, aspirate a volume of air equal to the medication dose from first medication (Vial A).	
___	___	___	4. Inject air into Vial A, being careful that the needle does not touch the solution.	
___	___	___	5. Remove syringe from Vial A.	
___	___	___	a. Aspirate volume of air equal to the medication dose from second medication (Vial B).	
___	___	___	b. Inject air into Vial B.	
___	___	___	6. Invert Vial B, and withdraw the required volume of medication into syringe. Expel all air bubbles, and withdraw needle from Vial B.	
___	___	___	7. Determine what the total combined volume of the two medications would measure on the syringe scale.	
___	___	___	8. Insert needle into Vial A, invert vial, and carefully withdraw required volume of medication (as in step 6).	
___	___	___	9. Withdraw needle from Vial A and replace needle guard.	
___	___	___	10. Check medication and dosage before returning or discarding vials. Label syringe with medication.	
			Modification for Insulin	
			Equipment	
___	___	___	1. Perform hand hygiene	
___	___	___	2. When preparing insulin in suspension, gently rotate vials between palms of hands to mix the suspension.	
___	___	___	3. Follow steps 2 through 10 as above.	
___	___	___	4. Establish a routine order for drawing up insulin. The shorter-acting regular insulin is drawn up first, followed by the cloudy intermediate-acting insulin. Glargine (Lantus), detemir (Levemir), and glulisine (Apidra) insulins cannot be mixed with other types of insulin.	

Procedure Checklist for Fundamentals of Nursing: Human Health and Function, 7th edition

Name ______________________ Date ______________________

Unit ______________________ Position ______________________

Instructor/Evaluator: ______________________ Position ______________________

PROCEDURE 19-6

Administering Intradermal Injections

Goal: Administer medication into the dermal tissue to screen for an allergic (antigen–antibody) dermal reaction, to screen for tuberculosis, or to administer local anesthesia.

Excellent	Satisfactory	Needs Practice		Comments
____	____	____	1. Check medication order. See Procedure 19-1, steps 1 through 6.	
____	____	____	2. Assemble needle and syringe.	
____	____	____	3. Remove needle guard and withdraw medication from vial (see Procedure 19-3).	
____	____	____	4. Identify patient by two identifiers (name, MRN, Social Security number, or birth date), checking identification bracelet. Scan bracelet if using BCMA. Repeat check of six rights.	
____	____	____	5. Close door or bed curtains and explain the procedure to the patient, then educate patient about medication.	
____	____	____	6. Don gloves. Select injection site that is relatively hairless and free from tenderness, swelling, scarring, and inflammation.	
____	____	____	7. Cleanse the site with an antimicrobial swab and then allow the skin to dry.	
____	____	____	8. Remove needle guard. Hold syringe in dominant hand. Gently pull skin distal to intended injection site taut with nondominant hand.	
____	____	____	9. Holding syringe from above, at a 10- to 15-degree angle (almost parallel to skin), gently insert needle, bevel up, about 1/8 inch until dermis barely covers bevel.	
____	____	____	10. Stabilize needle; inject medication slowly over 3 to 5 seconds while watching for a small wheal or blister to appear.	
____	____	____	11. Withdraw needle at the same angle at which it was inserted. Do not wipe or massage site.	
____	____	____	12. Do not recap needle. Dispose of syringe and needle in sharps container.	
____	____	____	13. Record time and site of injection according to best protocol.	
____	____	____	14. Instruct patient when to return for reading of response—15 to 60 minutes after injection for allergy testing and usually 48 to 72 hours after injection for TST.	

Procedure Checklist for Fundamentals of Nursing: Human Health and Function, 7th edition

Name ______________________ Date ______________________

Unit ______________________ Position ______________________

Instructor/Evaluator: ______________________ Position ______________________

PROCEDURE 19-7

Administering Subcutaneous Injections

Excellent	Satisfactory	Needs Practice	**Goal:** Ensure more rapid absorption and action of a drug than can be achieved orally; administer drugs to patients who are unable to take oral medications (e.g., unconscious, nausea/vomiting, NPO status); administer medications that are not active by the oral route or are inactivated by digestive enzymes (e.g., heparin, insulin).	**Comments**
____	____	____	1. Check medication order. Assess allergies. See Procedure 19-1, steps 1 through 6.	
____	____	____	2. Assemble needle and syringe.	
____	____	____	3. Remove needle guard and withdraw medication from container (see Procedures 19-3 and 19-4).	
____	____	____	4. Identify patient by two identifiers. Scan bracelet if using BCMA. Recheck six rights.	
____	____	____	5. Close door or bed curtains and explain the procedure to the patient, then educate patient about medication.	
____	____	____	6. Don gloves.	
____	____	____	7. Select an injection site that is free from tenderness, swelling, scarring, and inflammation.	
____	____	____	8. Cleanse site with antiseptic swab, using a circular motion from center toward outside. Allow area to dry thoroughly.	
____	____	____	9. Remove needle guard. Hold syringe in dominant hand. Place nondominant hand on either side of injection site. Spread or bunch skin to stabilize site and identify subcutaneous tissue.	
____	____	____	10. Hold syringe between thumb and forefinger of dominant hand (like a dart). Inject needle quickly at a 45- to 90-degree angle depending on the amount of subcutaneous tissue. Release bunched skin.	
____	____	____	11. Inject medication with slow, even pressure.	
____	____	____	12. Remove needle quickly at the same angle at which it was inserted while supporting the surrounding tissue with your nondominant hand. Apply gentle pressure to the site with a gauze square after the needle is withdrawn. Do not massage the site.	

Excellent	Satisfactory	Needs Practice	PROCEDURE 19-7 **Administering Subcutaneous Injections** *(Continued)*	Comments
____	____	____	13. Assist patient to a position of comfort.	
____	____	____	14. Do not recap needle. Activate the needle guard. Dispose of syringe and needle in sharps container.	
____	____	____	15. Perform hand hygiene.	
____	____	____	16. Document according to best protocol.	

Procedure Checklist for Fundamentals of Nursing: Human Health and Function, 7th edition

Name ____________________ Date ____________________

Unit ____________________ Position ____________________

Instructor/Evaluator: ____________________ Position ____________________

PROCEDURE 19-8

Administering Intramuscular Injections

Goal: Administer medication deeply into muscle tissue, without injury to the patient; administer a medication that requires absorption and onset of action quicker than the oral route without irritating the subcutaneous tissues.

Excellent	Satisfactory	Needs Practice		Comments
___	___	___	1. Check medication order. See Procedure 19-1, steps 1 through 6. Assemble needle and syringe.	
___	___	___	2. Prepare needle, syringe, and medication by following the appropriate steps in Procedures 19-3 or 19-4. If medication is known to be irritating to subcutaneous tissues, replace needle after withdrawing medication.	
___	___	___	3. Assess for allergies. Identify patient by two identifiers. Scan bracelet if using BCMA. Recheck six rights.	
___	___	___	4. Close door or bed curtains and explain the procedure to the patient, then educate patient about medication.	
___	___	___	5. Don gloves. Assist patient to a comfortable position, and expose only the area to be injected.	
___	___	___	6. Select appropriate injection site by inspecting muscle size and integrity. Consider volume of medication to be injected.	
___	___	___	7. Use anatomic landmarks to locate the exact injection site.	
___	___	___	8. Cleanse the site with antiseptic swab, wiping from center of site and rotating outward.	
___	___	___	9. Remove needle guard. Hold syringe between thumb and forefinger of dominant hand, like a dart. Spread skin at the site with nondominant hand. Encourage the patient to relax the muscle or use distraction techniques.	
___	___	___	10. Insert needle quickly at a 90-degree angle to the patient's skin surface.	
___	___	___	11. Stabilize syringe barrel by grasping with nondominant hand, if recommended (CDC, 2011). Slowly inject medication.	
___	___	___	12. Withdraw needle while pressing antiseptic swab above site.	
___	___	___	13. Apply gentle pressure at the site with dry gauze.	
___	___	___	14. Do not recap needle. Activate needle guard. Dispose of equipment in sharps container.	

PROCEDURE 19-8

Administering Intramuscular Injections *(Continued)*

Excellent	Satisfactory	Needs Practice		Comments
___	___	___	15. Perform hand hygiene.	
___	___	___	16. Record medication and patient response according to best protocol.	
			Variations for Z-Track Injection	
___	___	___	1. When preparing the injection site, pull the skin and subcutaneous tissues about 1 to 1.5 inches to one side of the selected site.	
___	___	___	2. Insert the syringe at a 90-degree angle. Do not release your nondominant hand that is stretching the skin to stabilize the syringe.	
___	___	___	3. Administer medication while continuing traction on skin.	
___	___	___	4. Leave needle inserted an additional 10 seconds.	
___	___	___	5. Simultaneously remove needle along the line of insertion and release traction on skin.	

Procedure Checklist for Fundamentals of Nursing: Human Health and Function, 7th edition

Name ______________________ Date ______________________

Unit ______________________ Position ______________________

Instructor/Evaluator: ______________________ Position ______________________

PROCEDURE 19-9

Administering Medications by Intravenous Bolus (less than 5 minutes)

Excellent	Satisfactory	Needs Practice	**Goal:** Achieve high blood levels of a medication in a short period; achieve immediate and maximal effects of a medication.	Comments
___	___	___	1. Check medication order. See Procedure 19-1, steps 1 through 6.	
___	___	___	2. If medication has not been prepared and labeled by pharmacy, the nurse prepares the medication. Draw up ordered medication from vial or ampule. Read package insert for proper amount and solution for dilution. Note rate of administration as well as compatibility with infusing IV solutions. Label syringe with patient's name, name of medication, and dose. Remove needle and dispose of it properly.	
___	___	___	3. Assess patient allergies. Identify the patient with two identifiers and recheck the six rights. Scan patient's identification bracelet if using BCMA.	
___	___	___	4. Close door or bed curtains and explain the procedure to the patient, then educate patient about medication.	
___	___	___	5. Assess IV site for signs of infiltration or phlebitis.	
___	___	___	6. Don clean gloves.	
			Administering Medication into an Existing Intravenous Line	
___	___	___	7. Select injection port or "Y" site in IV tubing closest to the IV insertion site. Clean port with antimicrobial swab.	
___	___	___	8. Uncap the syringe. Steady the port with your nondominant hand while inserting the needleless device into center of injection port.	
___	___	___	9. Occlude the tubing by folding it between your fingers (or using clamp).	
___	___	___	10. Pull back on plunger to assess for blood return.	
___	___	___	11. Inject the medication slowly into the IV port at the prescribed rate. It is helpful to use a watch to time the administration rate.	
___	___	___	12. If IV medication and IV solution in tubing are incompatible, flush line with normal saline solution while occluding catheter above port. Administer medication at prescribed rate; reflush with 10 mL of sterile normal saline solution and release occlusion.	

Excellent	Satisfactory	Needs Practice	PROCEDURE 19-9 **Administering Medications by Intravenous Bolus (less than 5 minutes)** *(Continued)*	
			Administering the Drug Into an Intermittent Infusion Device or Lock Device	
___	___	___	7. Clean port with antimicrobial swab using friction.	
___	___	___	8. Stabilize port with your nondominant hand and insert syringe with 1 mL normal saline solution into injection port.	
___	___	___	9. Release the clamp on the extension tubing of the medication lock. Optional: Aspirate gently and check for blood return.	
___	___	___	10. Gently flush with normal saline by pushing slowly on the syringe plunger. Observe the insertion site while inserting the saline. Remove the syringe.	
___	___	___	11. Insert syringe with medication into injection port. Inject medication slowly at the prescribed rate. Use watch to time administration rate. Remove syringe. Do not force the injection if resistance is felt.	
___	___	___	12. Insert syringe with 1 to 3 mL of normal saline into injection port and gently flush the port with saline. To gain positive pressure, clamp the IV tubing as you are still flushing the last of the saline into the medication lock. Remove the syringe from the injection port.	
___	___	___	13. Dispose of used syringes properly, remove gloves, and wash hands.	
___	___	___	14. Document medication administration.	
___	___	___	15. Evaluate and chart the patient's response to medication therapy and document according to agency policy.	

Procedure Checklist for Fundamentals of Nursing: Human Health and Function, 7th edition

Name ______________________ Date ______________________

Unit ______________________ Position ______________________

Instructor/Evaluator: ______________________ Position ______________________

PROCEDURE 20-1
Initiating Intravenous Therapy

Excellent	Satisfactory	Needs Practice	**Goal:** To maintain or replace fluids for daily body fluid requirements; to provide electrolytes to maintain or restore electrolyte balance; to deliver glucose and nutrients for use as an energy source; to deliver medication or blood products.	Comments
___	___	___	1. Verify the physician's order for IV therapy including solution type, amount, additives, and infusion rate.	
___	___	___	2. Gather all equipment and bring it to the patient's bedside.	
___	___	___	3. Perform hand hygiene.	
___	___	___	4. Identify the patient using two separate identifiers.	
___	___	___	5. Close door or bed curtains and explain the procedure to the patient.	
			Preparing the Solution	
___	___	___	6. Remove the IV solution bag from the outer plastic covering. Open all other equipment packages, maintaining sterility of the equipment.	
___	___	___	7. Grasp the IV administration set and close the flow clamp on the tubing. Attach an extension set tubing to the administration set if necessary.	
___	___	___	8. Remove the protective cap or tear the tab from the tubing insertion port on the solution container; remove the protective covering from the spike on the administration tubing. Hold the port carefully and firmly with one hand, then quickly insert the spike into the port with the other hand.	
___	___	___	9. Invert the solution container and hang it on the IV pole with the infusion pump. Compress the drip chamber until it is approximately half full. Remove the protective cap from the end of the infusion tubing (or extension set, if used); direct the end of the tubing toward a receptacle. Open the flow clamp on the tubing and allow the fluid to run through the tubing until all the air has been removed and the entire length of the tubing is filled with solution; then close the flow clamp.	
___	___	___	10. Attach the solution and tubing to the infusion control device according to the manufacturer's instructions. Apply label to the solution container if one has not already been applied by the pharmacy.	

Excellent	Satisfactory	Needs Practice	PROCEDURE 20-1 **Initiating Intravenous Therapy** *(Continued)*	Comments
			Selecting the Insertion Site	
___	___	___	6. Place the patient in a comfortable, reclining position, leaving the arm in a dependent position. Place a towel or protective pad under the extremity to be used. Inspect and palpate the patient's extremity to identify an appropriate vein. Select the puncture site. If long-term therapy is anticipated, start with a vein at the most distal site so that you can move proximally as needed for subsequent IV insertion sites.	
___	___	___	7. Put on clean gloves and apply a tourniquet about 6 inches (15 cm) above the intended puncture site. Ensure that the ends of the tourniquet are positioned away from the intended insertion site. Check for a radial pulse. If it isn't present, release the tourniquet and reapply it with less tension.	
___	___	___	8. Lightly palpate the vein with the index and middle fingers of your nondominant hand. Stretch the skin to anchor the vein. If the vein feels hard or ropelike, select another site.	
			Inserting the Device and Initiating Therapy	
___	___	___	6. Administer a local anesthetic according to agency policy (e.g., 0.1 to 0.2 mL lidocaine 1% without epinephrine injected intradermally). If a transdermal analgesic cream (EMLA) is ordered, ensure adequate time from the application of the topical agent to insertion.	
___	___	___	7. Clean the site using the approved antimicrobial agent (chlorhexidine gluconate or povidone-iodine) according to facility policy. Work in a circular motion outward from the site to a diameter of 2 to 4 inches (5 to 10 cm), and allow the agent to dry. If facility policy permits, clip hair around the intended insertion site for a distance of up to 2 inches. Do not shave or use depilatory creams, which may injure the skin and increase risk of infection.	
___	___	___	8. Grasp the device. Using the thumb of your nondominant hand, stretch the skin taut below the puncture site. If using a vein in the hand, position the hand in a slightly flexed position to keep the skin taut. Tell the patient that you are about to insert the device and that you need him or her to remain still.	

Excellent	Satisfactory	Needs Practice	PROCEDURE 20-1 **Initiating Intravenous Therapy** *(Continued)*	Comments
___	___	___	9. Hold the needle bevel up at a 15- to 30-degree angle, depending on estimated depth of the vein, and enter the skin parallel to the vein. Decrease the angle of the needle until almost parallel with the skin, and advance the device into the vein in one motion either from directly over the vein or from the side. You will feel a sense of release or a pop as you enter the vein. Check for blood return and then advance the device, maintaining the device parallel to the skin until the hub is at the insertion site.	
___	___	___	10. Hold finger pressure over end of catheter while removing needle stylet.	
___	___	___	11. Remove the tourniquet quickly. While holding the hub with your nondominant hand, attach the end of the infusion tubing to the device.	
			Applying a Dressing	
___	___	___	6. Apply a dressing (most commonly a transparent, semipermeable dressing) to the site. Alternatively, secure the device with nonallergenic tape and cover with a 2 × 2 gauze.	
___	___	___	7. Loop any IV tubing on the patient's extremity and secure with tape.	
___	___	___	8. Label the dressing with the date and time of insertion; device type, gauge, and size; and your initials.	
___	___	___	9. Begin the infusion, setting the infusion pump to the prescribed rate of flow. Assess the flow of the solution and infusion control device function. Inspect the site for signs of infiltration.	
			Providing Ongoing Care	
___	___	___	6. Dispose of all equipment and remove gloves. Perform hand hygiene.	
___	___	___	7. Apply site protection device and secure as necessary.	
___	___	___	8. Assist the patient to a comfortable position. Assess the patient's tolerance of the procedure.	
___	___	___	9. Document the procedure, including the date and time of the venipuncture; device type, gauge, and length; location of insertion site and appearance; type and flow rate of the IV solution; patient's response (including adverse reactions); patient teaching performed; and patient's understanding of the teaching.	
___	___	___	10. Monitor infusion rate, condition of IV site, and patient complaints, initially approximately 30 minutes after beginning the infusion and then according to facility policy. Change dressing, tubing, and solutions according to facility policy.	

Procedure Checklist for Fundamentals of Nursing: Human Health and Function, 7th edition

Name ______________________ Date ______________

Unit ______________________ Position ______________

Instructor/Evaluator: ______________________ Position ______________

PROCEDURE 20-2

Monitoring an Intravenous Infusion

Excellent	Satisfactory	Needs Practice	**Goal:** Provide a safe, patent route for infusion of IV therapy; ensure correct infusion of IV fluids; detect IV complications promptly.	**Comments**
____	____	____	1. Perform hand hygiene.	
____	____	____	2. Identify the patient using two separate identifiers.	
____	____	____	3. Close door or bed curtains and explain the procedure to the patient.	
____	____	____	4. Compare IV fluid currently infusing with the ordered solution.	
____	____	____	5. Inspect the rate of flow at least every hour. For gravity-regulated IVs, check actual flow rate for 15 seconds and multiply by 4 for the minute rate. Compare the assessed rate with prescribed flow rate. If the infusion is ahead of schedule, slow it so the infusion will complete at the planned time. If infusion is behind schedule, review hospital policy and complete patient assessment before increasing flow rate; some agencies require a physician's order to increase the rate of flow. If EID is used, the hourly infusion rate in milliliters per hour is programmed into the machine.	
____	____	____	6. Inspect the system for leakage; if present, locate the source. Tighten all connections within the system. If leak persists, slow the IV flow rate to keep the vein open and replace tubing with sterile set.	
____	____	____	7. Inspect the tubing for kinks or blockages. Loosely coil tubing and place it on the bed.	
____	____	____	8. Inspect the insertion site and dressing for leakage of IV solution.	
____	____	____	9. Inspect the infusion site for infiltration. Infiltration occurs when the needle becomes dislodged from the vein and IV fluid flows into the interstitial tissue. Look for signs of infiltration, including decreased flow rate, swelling, pallor, coolness, and discomfort at or above needle insertion site. If signs are present, change the IV site. If a large amount of fluid has infiltrated, elevate the arm above the heart on several pillows.	

Excellent	Satisfactory	Needs Practice	PROCEDURE 20-2 **Monitoring an Intravenous Infusion** *(Continued)*	Comments
___	___	___	10. Inspect arm above the insertion point for signs of phlebitis, including redness, swelling, warmth, and pain along the vein above IV insertion site. If present, discontinue the IV and restart in another area. Ask the patient to report burning or pain at the IV site. If you suspect phlebitis is present, notify the IV team or physician and check agency policy for treating phlebitis.	
___	___	___	11. Inspect the insertion site for bleeding.	
___	___	___	12. Inspect the site for local manifestations of infection including redness, pus, warmth, induration, and pain. Inspect the patient for systemic manifestations of infection, including chills, fever, tachycardia, and hypotension, that may accompany local infection. Inspect the patient for additional complications of IV therapy (e.g., fluid overload).	
___	___	___	13. Check EID alarm settings. Attend to all alarms in a timely manner.	
___	___	___	14. Although monitoring IV therapy is a nursing responsibility, if the patient is able to comply, teach him or her to contact the nurse if the following occur:	
___	___	___	a. The flow rate changes suddenly	
___	___	___	b. The fluid container is almost empty	
___	___	___	c. Blood is in the tubing	
___	___	___	d. The site becomes uncomfortable	
___	___	___	15. Chart any findings indicating complications of IV therapy (e.g., infiltration).	

Procedure Checklist for Fundamentals of Nursing: Human Health and Function, 7th edition

Name ______________________ Date ______________________

Unit ______________________ Position ______________________

Instructor/Evaluator: ______________________ Position ______________________

PROCEDURE 20-3

Peripheral IV Site Care

Excellent	Satisfactory	Needs Practice	**Goal:** Protect the IV site from infection; permit visual inspection of the IV site to promptly detect complications of therapy.	**Comments**
____	____	____	1. Perform hand hygiene	
____	____	____	2. Identify the patient.	
____	____	____	3. Close door or bed curtains and explain the procedure to the patient.	
____	____	____	4. Put on clean gloves. Place waterproof pad under IV site.	
____	____	____	5. Inspect site for signs of infection, infiltration, and thrombophlebitis.	
____	____	____	6. Hold catheter in place with your nondominant hand and gently remove dressing and tape. For transparent dressing, gently stretch the film horizontal to the skin.	
____	____	____	7. Clean the entry site with a chlorhexidine solution, using a circular motion and moving from the center outward. Allow the area to dry completely; do not blow or blot dry.	
____	____	____	8. Attach new nonsuture securing device, using extreme care to not dislodge catheter. Apply transparent semipermeable dressing to the IV site. Take care not to tape over the IV connection or IV tubing.	
____	____	____	9. Label dressing with date, time, and initials. Secure IV tubing with additional tape if necessary.	
____	____	____	10. Assess IV flow is accurate and system is patent.	
____	____	____	11. Remove gloves and perform hand hygiene. Document dressing change and observations.	

Procedure Checklist for Fundamentals of Nursing: Human Health and Function, 7th edition

Name ______________________ Date ______________

Unit ______________________ Position ______________

Instructor/Evaluator: ______________________ Position ______________

PROCEDURE 20-4

Peripherally Inserted Central Venous Access Device (PICC) Site Care

Goal: Protect the PICC site from infection; permit visual inspection of the PICC site to promptly detect complications of therapy.

Excellent	Satisfactory	Needs Practice		Comments
___	___	___	1. Perform hand hygiene.	
___	___	___	2. Identify the patient.	
___	___	___	3. Close door or bed curtains and explain the procedure to the patient.	
___	___	___	4. Place patient in a comfortable position.	
___	___	___	5. Apply mask. Have patient put on mask and turn head away from site. Prepare sterile field and place sterile drape around site.	
___	___	___	6. Assess insertion site for infection and phlebitis.	
___	___	___	7. Put on clean gloves. Stabilize catheter with thumb. Remove old dressing, stretching horizontally and then working proximally. Carefully remove securing device. Remove gloves.	
___	___	___	8. Don sterile gloves and clean the area around the site with a chlorhexidine solution. Move in a circular fashion, cleaning from the insertion site outward 2 to 3 inches. Allow to dry; do not blow or blot.	
___	___	___	9. Re-dress the site with a transparent semipermeable dressing, according to agency policy. Secure tubing and all Luer lock connections.	
___	___	___	10. Label the dressing with date, time, and initials.	
___	___	___	11. Clamp all lines of device and remove injection caps. Cleanse catheter ends with antimicrobial swab and reapply new injection caps.	
___	___	___	12. Flush the catheter according to agency policy using a 10-cc syringe. Use the "pulse-pause" technique, always ending with positive pressure by clamping prior to ending the flush.	
___	___	___	13. Discard all used items properly. Reposition the patient comfortably. Document dressing change and observations.	

Procedure Checklist for Fundamentals of Nursing: Human Health and Function, 7th edition

Name ______________________ Date ______________

Unit ______________________ Position ______________

Instructor/Evaluator: ______________________ Position ______________

PROCEDURE 20-5

Changing Intravenous Solution and Tubing

Excellent	Satisfactory	Needs Practice	**Goal:** Deliver IV therapy as ordered; decrease risk of patient infection.	Comments
___	___	___	1. Perform hand hygiene.	
___	___	___	2. Identify the patient.	
___	___	___	3. Close door or bed curtains and explain the procedure to the patient.	
			Changing Solution Container	
___	___	___	4. Compare solution with physician's order. Assess patient allergies. Adhere to six rights of medication administration, including identifying the patient with two separate identifiers.	
___	___	___	5. Remove IV bag from outer wrapper. Look for leaks or impurities in the bag and check the IV fluid bag for expiration date.	
___	___	___	6. Label solution container with patient's name, solution type, additives, date, and time hung. If labeled by pharmacy, check prelabeled container with physician's order. Record solution change in the patient's record.	
___	___	___	7. Prepare container for spiking:	
___	___	___	a. If solution is in a plastic bag, remove plastic cover from entry nipple. Maintain sterility of nipple end.	
___	___	___	b. If solution is in a bottle, remove metal cap, metal disk, and rubber disk. Maintain sterility of bottle top.	
___	___	___	8. Close the clamp on the existing tubing. If using an electronic device, turn the device to the "hold" position.	
___	___	___	9. Take old solution container from pole and invert it. Quickly remove spike from used container, maintaining spike sterility.	
___	___	___	10. Spike new IV container with firm push/twist motion and hang new container on IV pole. Alternatively, you can hang the IV bag, then spike the new container.	
___	___	___	11. Inspect tubing for air bubbles, and assess that drip chamber is half full of solution.	
___	___	___	12. Reopen and adjust clamp to regulate flow rate or program EID, according to orders.	

Excellent	Satisfactory	Needs Practice	PROCEDURE 20-5 **Changing Intravenous Solution and Tubing** *(Continued)*	Comments
			Changing Intravenous Tubing Connected Directly Into the Hub of the Intravenous Access Catheter	
___	___	___	1. Follow steps 1 through 6 of the Changing Solution Container section.	
___	___	___	2. Open new tubing package. Keep protective covers on spike and catheter adaptor.	
___	___	___	3. Adjust roller clamp on new tubing to fully closed position.	
___	___	___	4. Prepare new solution container as directed in step 5 of the Changing Solution Container section.	
___	___	___	5. Maintaining sterility, remove protective cover from spike and insert spike into new solution container.	
___	___	___	6. Hang container and "prime" drip chamber by squeezing gently, allowing to fill half full.	
___	___	___	7. Remove protective cap from end of IV tubing, and adjust roller clamp to flush tubing with fluid. Replace protective cap.	
___	___	___	8. Adjust roller clamp on old tubing to close fully.	
___	___	___	9. Place towel or disposable pad under extremity. Don clean, disposable gloves.	
___	___	___	10. Hold catheter hub with fingers of one hand (may use hemostat). With other hand, loosen old tubing using gentle twisting motion. (*Note:* The dressing may have to be removed.)	
___	___	___	11. Cleanse cap with antiseptic swab using friction. Grasp new tubing, remove protective catheter cap, disconnect IV tubing, and Luer lock new tubing tightly into needle hub while continuing to stabilize catheter hub with other hand.	
___	___	___	12. Insert cassette into EID. Program the EID or adjust roller clamp to start solution flowing according to physician's order.	
___	___	___	13. Discard gloves.	
___	___	___	14. Secure tubing with tape.	
___	___	___	15. If dressing was removed, apply new dressing to IV site according to agency policy.	
___	___	___	16. Label new tubing with date, time, and your initials.	
___	___	___	17. Label solution container with patient's name, solution type, additives, and date and time hung (if not already done). Record solution and tubing change.	

Procedure Checklist for Fundamentals of Nursing: Human Health and Function, 7th edition

Name ________________ Date ________________

Unit ________________ Position ________________

Instructor/Evaluator: ________________ Position ________________

PROCEDURE 20-6

Converting to an Intermittent Infusion Device and Flushing

Excellent	Satisfactory	Needs Practice	**Goal:** Maintain patency of IVs used intermittently for medication and emergency IV access; permits patient increased mobility and freedom if continuous IV infusion is not required.	**Comments**
___	___	___	1. Perform hand hygiene.	
___	___	___	2. Identify the patient.	
___	___	___	3. Close door or bed curtains and explain the procedure to the patient.	
___	___	___	4. Assess IV site for signs of phlebitis, infiltration, or infection. If complications are detected, discontinue the IV and restart it in another site.	
___	___	___	5. Prepare 10-mL syringe with 3 mL of NaCl (or heparin flush solution according to agency policy or manufacturer recommendations for specific intravascular device). Prefilled 10-mL NaCl syringes are preferred to decrease risk of contamination. Label syringes if not using prelabeled syringe.	
			Converting to an IID When Extension Tubing Is in Place	
___	___	___	6. Clamp off primary IV tubing.	
___	___	___	7. Put on clean gloves. Clamp the extension tubing. Disconnect IV tubing from extension tubing.	
___	___	___	8. Cleanse port on extension tubing with antiseptic swab using friction for 15 seconds.	
___	___	___	9. Unclamp the extension set and insert a normal saline or heparin flush syringe into the cap. Flush according to agency policy. Inject the recommended amount of solution using pulsating technique, ending with 0.5 cc of solution remaining in syringe. Do not force if resistance is met. Reclamp the extension tubing and remove the syringe. (*Note:* This procedure must be done at least every 8 hours or after each use of the catheter for IV medications to ensure catheter patency. Most agencies recommend changing IV locks every 72 hours to ensure patency and to prevent common complications of IV therapy.)	

PROCEDURE 20-6

Converting to an Intermittent Infusion Device and Flushing *(Continued)*

Excellent	Satisfactory	Needs Practice		Comments
____	____	____	10. Dispose of syringes in proper container. Remove gloves and dispose of them properly.	
____	____	____	11. Tape adaptor device and extension tubing.	
____	____	____	12. Perform hand hygiene.	
____	____	____	13. Document date, time, route, amount, and type of flush solution. Also document assessment of site.	

Procedure Checklist for Fundamentals of Nursing: Human Health and Function, 7th edition

Name ______________________ Date ______________________

Unit ______________________ Position ______________________

Instructor/Evaluator: ______________________ Position ______________________

PROCEDURE 20-7

Administering Intravenous Medications Using Intermittent Infusion Technique

Excellent	Satisfactory	Needs Practice	**Goal:** Maintain therapeutic levels of medication in patient's blood; dilute irritating IV medications; prevent complications associated with bolus administration by delivering medications over a longer period; prevent combining incompatible medications.	**Comments**
____	____	____	1. Check medication order. See Procedure 19-1, steps 1 through 6.	
			Administering IV Medications When Using Syringe Pump and Intermittent Infusion Device	
____	____	____	2. Prepare the medication syringe and IV tubing. Examine the syringe for any air bubbles and expel any that are present. Attach the syringe to the extension tubing, and gently push the syringe plunger to prime the tubing. Cover adaptor.	
____	____	____	3. Secure the medication syringe into the pump with the flange of the syringe in the clamp's groove.	
____	____	____	4. Assess for patient allergies. Confirm the patient's identity by checking two separate identifiers. Scan the patient's bracelet if using bar code medication administration. Recheck the six rights and explain the procedure to the patient.	
____	____	____	5. Assess the IV site for inflammation or infiltration.	
____	____	____	6. Don gloves.	
____	____	____	7. Attach syringe with normal saline into the lock device. Flush lock with normal saline.	
____	____	____	8. Attach tubing to lock device. Secure IV tubing to IV site with tape.	
____	____	____	9. Program the pump for the appropriate infusion speed and press the start key. The medication syringe label often indicates the suggested infusion speed, typically 30 to 60 minutes. If uncertain, consult a drug reference handbook or pharmacist.	
____	____	____	10. Document medication administration.	
____	____	____	11. Assess the patient and infusion device 5 to 10 minutes after infusion has begun.	
____	____	____	12. When the completion alarm sounds, return to patient's room and press the pump's stop key.	

Excellent	Satisfactory	Needs Practice	PROCEDURE 20-7 **Administering Intravenous Medications Using Intermittent Infusion Technique** *(Continued)*	Comments
___	___	___	13. Don gloves. Remove tubing from lock device. Attach syringe with 1 to 3 mL of normal saline and flush lock using push pulse technique ending with positive pressure.	
___	___	___	14. Replace lock with new sterile cap.	
___	___	___	15. Dispose of syringes in proper container. Perform hand hygiene.	
			Administering Intermittent IV Medication Into Primary IV Line Using an Electronic Infusion Device (EID) or Smart Pump	
			Equipment	
___	___	___	1. Check medication order. See Procedure 19-1, steps 1 through 6. Prepare medication, tubing, and EID according to procedures described earlier.	
___	___	___	2. Assess patient allergies. Confirm patient's identity using two identifiers and check six rights again.	
___	___	___	3. Assess the IV site for inflammation or infiltration.	
___	___	___	4. Position infusion bags so that the medication (secondary) bag is at or above the level of the primary IV solution. Insert secondary line into the adaptor port.	
___	___	___	5. Check compatibility of medications to be administered with the IV solution being infused and any other infusing medications. If medication is not compatible with primary IV solution, clamp primary IV tubing above injection port, attach syringe with 20-mL of normal saline flush solution, and flush IV line. Do not administer IV medication through tubing that is infusing blood products or TPN.	
___	___	___	6. Clean the access port on the primary IV infusion tubing using an antimicrobial swab.	
___	___	___	7. Connect secondary (piggyback) line to injection port or Y-site on IV tubing closest to IV insertion site.	
___	___	___	8. Program the EID or smart pump with the correct volume and infusion rate for secondary infusion. Release clamps and press start button.	
___	___	___	9. When medication has infused, clamp tubing and leave attached. Discard medication bag and tubing if last dose or if tubing will need to be changed before the next dose. Do not loop tubing together at Y-port.	
___	___	___	10. Perform hand hygiene.	
___	___	___	11. Document medication administration and add IV volume to IV intake.	

Procedure Checklist for Fundamentals of Nursing: Human Health and Function, 7th edition

Name ______________________ Date ______________

Unit ______________________ Position ______________

Instructor/Evaluator: ______________________ Position ______________

PROCEDURE 20-8

Monitoring Total Parenteral Nutrition and Administering Intralipids

Excellent	Satisfactory	Needs Practice	**Goal:** Provide parenteral nutritional support to malnourished patients; provide parenteral nutritional support to patients who are NPO for extended periods of time; provide parenteral nutritional support to patients requiring bypass of the gastrointestinal tract for prolonged periods; provide parenteral nutritional support to patients who have excessive metabolic needs due to trauma, cancer, or hypermetabolic states.	**Comments**
____	____	____	1. Perform hand hygiene.	
____	____	____	2. Identify the patient using two separate identifiers.	
____	____	____	3. Close door or bed curtains and explain the procedure to the patient.	
			Monitoring Total Parenteral Nutrition Therapy	
____	____	____	4. Schedule and assist patient with chest x-ray after central catheter insertion.	
____	____	____	5. Confirm correct solution against physician's order. Check solution's expiration date. Assess patient allergies. Set the EID for the proper infusion rate. (*Note:* Solutions with more than 10% dextrose must be infused directly into a central catheter to rapidly dilute the solution and prevent thrombophlebitis. Constant flow rate helps prevent hyperglycemia and electrolyte imbalances.)	
____	____	____	6. Inspect tubing and catheter connection for leaks or kinks. Tape all connections. Change tubing every 24 hours according to agency policy.	
____	____	____	7. Inspect insertion site for infiltration, thrombophlebitis, or drainage. If present, notify physician. The physician may order removal of the catheter and culture of the catheter tip.	
____	____	____	8. Monitor vital signs, including temperature, every 4 hours.	
____	____	____	9. Use the TPN line only for administration of TPN and lipids. Do not use the line for any other reason.	
____	____	____	10. Monitor patient's blood glucose as ordered (usually every 6 to 12 hours). Notify physician if abnormal.	
____	____	____	11. Monitor laboratory tests of electrolytes, blood urea nitrogen (BUN), and glucose, as ordered, and report abnormal findings.	

Excellent	Satisfactory	Needs Practice	PROCEDURE 20-8 **Monitoring Total Parenteral Nutrition and Administering Intralipids** *(Continued)*	Comments
___	___	___	12. Maintain accurate record of intake and output to monitor fluid balance.	
___	___	___	13. Weigh patient daily and record.	
___	___	___	14. Inspect dressing once a shift for drainage and intactness. Change dressing whenever loose or moist, and perform site care at least every 48 hours.	
			Administering Intralipids	
___	___	___	1. Check solution against physician's order. Inspect solution for separation of emulsion into layers or for froth. Do not use if present.	
___	___	___	2. Assess patient allergies to egg yolks or soy products.	
___	___	___	3. Attach fat emulsion tubing to bottle. Prime tubing as for a conventional IV.	
___	___	___	4. Identify patient using two separate identifiers. Adhere to the six rights of medication administration.	
___	___	___	5. Identify Y-port on tubing (below in-line filter). Cleanse Y-port with antiseptic swab. Allow to dry. Insert connector into port. Secure with tape. (*Note:* Lipids can be infused into a peripheral IV.)	
___	___	___	6. Adjust flow rate to infuse at 1.0 mL per minute for adults and 0.1 mL per minute for children. Infuse at this rate for 30 minutes while monitoring the patient and vital signs.	
___	___	___	7. If no adverse reactions occur, adjust flow rate:	
___	___	___	a. *Adults:* 500 mL intralipid over 4 to 6 hours, or as ordered.	
___	___	___	b. *Children:* Up to 1 g per kilogram over 4 hours.	

Procedure Checklist for Fundamentals of Nursing: Human Health and Function, 7th edition

Name ______________________ Date ______________________

Unit ______________________ Position ______________________

Instructor/Evaluator: ______________________ Position ______________________

PROCEDURE 20-9
Administering a Blood Transfusion

Excellent	Satisfactory	Needs Practice	**Goal**: Replace blood volume or blood components lost through trauma, surgery, or a disease process; prevent complications from transfusing incompatible blood products.	**Comments**
___	___	___	1. Perform hand hygiene.	
___	___	___	2. Identify the patient using two separate identifiers.	
___	___	___	3. Close door or bed curtains and explain the procedure to the patient.	
___	___	___	4. Ensure informed consent has been signed by provider and patient. Teach patient what to report in the event of an adverse reaction, such as chills, back pain, headache, nausea or vomiting, rapid heart rate, rapid breathing, or skin rash.	
___	___	___	5. Administer premedications, such as diphenhydramine (Benadryl), if ordered.	
___	___	___	6. Obtain patient's vital signs, including temperature.	
___	___	___	7. With another RN, a physician, or other licensed staff member at the patient's bedside, verify the blood component and the patient's identity by comparing the laboratory blood record with the following:	
___	___	___	a. The patient's name and identification number, both verbally and against patient's identification band	
___	___	___	b. The blood unit number on the blood bag label	
___	___	___	c. The blood ABO group and Rh factor on the blood bag label	
___	___	___	d. The type of blood component and the expiration date on the blood label.	
___	___	___	8. Inspect blood product for integrity of bag and appearance of component (clots, cloudiness, abnormal color). Note expiration date and time on the transfusion report.	
___	___	___	9. Wash your hands. Put on clean gloves.	
___	___	___	10. Open Y-type blood administration set, and clamp both rollers completely.	
___	___	___	11. Spike blood component unit bag port. Prime drip chamber and tubing with blood component.	
___	___	___	12. Spike 0.9% NaCl container with second spike. Keep roller clamp shut.	

PROCEDURE 20-9

Administering a Blood Transfusion *(Continued)*

Excellent	Satisfactory	Needs Practice		Comments
___	___	___	13. Remove primary IV tubing from catheter hub, and cover end with sterile protector.	
___	___	___	14. Attach blood administration tubing to catheter hub, and secure with tape. The IV should be started into an 18- or 19-gauge catheter.	
___	___	___	15. Open clamp to blood component. Open roller clamp below drip chamber and begin transfusion. Program EID to infuse blood slowly for first 15 minutes.	
___	___	___	16. Observe and document patient's condition during first 15 minutes, assessing for chilling, back pain, headache, nausea or vomiting, tachycardia, hypotension, tachypnea, fluid overload, or skin rash. (*Note:* If any adverse reactions occur, close clamp to blood, open clamp to 0.9% NaCl, and notify physician immediately. Follow agency policy for laboratory notification and obtaining blood and urine specimens.)	
___	___	___	17. If no adverse reactions occur after 15 minutes, reprogram EID to increase infusion according to physician's orders. A unit of RBCs is usually administered over 2 to 4 hours. Observe the patient for signs and symptoms of transfusion reaction at least every 30 minutes throughout the transfusion. Obtain vital signs when observations warrant. Document observations, including the absence of any signs of transfusion reaction, in the medical record.	
___	___	___	18. When blood transfusion is complete, clamp roller to blood and open roller to 0.9% NaCl. Infuse until tubing is clear (usually no more than 50 mL of normal saline).	
___	___	___	19. Obtain and document vital signs.	
___	___	___	20. If second blood component unit is to be transfused, slow 0.9% NaCl to keep vein open until next unit is available. Follow verification procedure and vital sign monitoring for each unit.	
___	___	___	21. If transfusion orders are complete, disconnect the blood administration tubing from the IV catheter hub. Reconnect the primary IV solution and tubing and adjust to desired rate.	
___	___	___	22. Wash hands and document procedure.	

Procedure Checklist for Fundamentals of Nursing: Human Health and Function, 7th edition

Name ______________________ Date ______________________

Unit ______________________ Position ______________________

Instructor/Evaluator: ______________________ Position ______________________

PROCEDURE 22-1

Application of Physical Restraints

Excellent	Satisfactory	Needs Practice	**Goal:** Prevent the patient from pulling out tubes or lines that could cause harm to the patient or negatively impact treatment; manage violent or self-destructive behavior that jeopardizes the immediate physical safety of the patient, staff members, or others.	**Comments**
____	____	____	1. Perform hand hygiene.	
____	____	____	2. Identify the patient.	
____	____	____	3. Close door or bed curtains and explain the procedure to the patient and patient's family.	
____	____	____	4. Select the appropriate restraint for the patient.	
			Wrist (or Ankle) Restraint	
____	____	____	5. Wrap the restraint around extremity with soft pad touching skin.	
____	____	____	6. Secure in place by fastening Velcro and or buckle. Ensure that two fingers can be inserted between the restraint and the patient's wrist.	
			Mitt Restraint	
____	____	____	6. Slide patient's hand into mitt restraint. Fingers do not need to go to the tip of the glove. Secure in place by fastening strap and Velcro around the narrowest part of the wrist. Ensure that two fingers can be inserted between the restraint and the patient's wrist. Sometimes a mitt restraint can be secured with a wrist restraint to the bed frame, but often mitts are used independently to prevent use of hands to grab.	
			Vest (Jacket) Restraint	
____	____	____	3. Select the correct size of vest noting back versus front of the restraint. Apply front of vest to front of patient and zip closed. Make sure you can slip fingers of your hand between the vest and the patient's abdomen.	
____	____	____	4. Fasten quick-release buckle to the bed springs or frame, never to the mattress or the bed rails.	

PROCEDURE 22-1

Application of Physical Restraints *(Continued)*

Excellent	Satisfactory	Needs Practice		Comments
___	___	___	5. Observe patients in restraints frequently and document according to policy, describing the patient's behavior, the intervention used, and the patient's response to the intervention. The patient must be assessed face-to-face within 1 hour of application and frequently thereafter.	
___	___	___	6. Remove the restraints at least every 2 hours and more often if necessary. Allow for ADLs.	

Procedure Checklist for Fundamentals of Nursing: Human Health and Function, 7th edition

Name ____________________ Date ____________________

Unit ____________________ Position ____________________

Instructor/Evaluator: ____________________ Position ____________________

PROCEDURE 23-1

Assisting With the Bath or Shower

Excellent	Satisfactory	Needs Practice	**Goal:** Cleanse the skin, control body odors, and promote self-esteem; stimulate circulation; provide an opportunity to assess skin and physical mobility; provide range-of-motion exercises for joints; promote relaxation and comfort.	**Comments**
____	____	____	1. Perform hand hygiene.	
____	____	____	2. Identify the patient.	
____	____	____	3. Close door or bed curtains and explain the procedure to the patient and patient's family.	
____	____	____	4. Make sure the tub or shower is clean.	
____	____	____	5. Prepare bathroom by placing towel or disposable bathmat on floor by tub or shower.	
____	____	____	6. Accompany or transport patient to the bathroom. Some patients may need to use a shower chair for transportation or support.	
____	____	____	7. Place "occupied" sign on door.	
____	____	____	8. Keep patient covered with a bath blanket until water is ready.	
____	____	____	9. Fill bathtub halfway with warm water (105°F [40.6°C]). Test water or have patient test water. If the patient is taking a shower, turn on shower and adjust water temperature.	
____	____	____	10. Help patient into shower or tub, providing necessary assistance.	
____	____	____	11. Instruct the patient in use of safety bars and call-light signal. Patient may prefer to sit in shower chair to prevent fatigue.	
____	____	____	12. If the patient is unable to shower independently, stay with the patient at all times. (Two nurses may be necessary for some patients.) Use handheld shower to wet patient. Wash patient with soap and washcloth using long, firm strokes.	
____	____	____	13. If patient is showering or bathing independently, check on patient within 15 minutes. Wash any areas that he or she could not reach.	
____	____	____	14. Assist with drying. Help patient out of tub or shower. If patient is unsteady, drain water before helping patient out of tub.	

PROCEDURE 23-1

Assisting With the Bath or Shower *(Continued)*

Excellent	Satisfactory	Needs Practice		Comments
____	____	____	15. Assist patient with dressing and grooming.	
____	____	____	16. Help patient to room. Return to bathroom and clean tub or shower according to agency policy. Discard soiled linen. Place "unoccupied" sign on door.	
____	____	____	17. Document procedure.	

Procedure Checklist for Fundamentals of Nursing: Human Health and Function, 7th edition

Name ______________________ Date ______________________

Unit ______________________ Position ______________________

Instructor/Evaluator: ______________________ Position ______________________

PROCEDURE 23-2

Bathing a Patient in Bed

Excellent	Satisfactory	Needs Practice	**Goal**: Cleanse the skin, control body odors, and promote self-esteem; stimulate circulation; provide an opportunity to assess skin and physical mobility; provide range-of-motion exercises for joints; promote relaxation and comfort.	**Comments**
____	____	____	1. Identify the patient.	
____	____	____	2. Close door or bed curtains and explain the procedure to the patient and patient's family.	
____	____	____	3. Help patient use bedpan, urinal, or commode if needed.	
____	____	____	4. Close window and door to decrease drafts.	
____	____	____	5. Perform hand hygiene.	
____	____	____	6. Raise bed to high position. Lock up side rail on opposite side of bed from your work.	
____	____	____	7. Remove top sheet and bedspread, then place bath blanket on patient. Help patient move closer to you. If top linen is to be reused, place it on back of chair; otherwise, place it in laundry bag.	
____	____	____	8. Lay towel across patient's chest.	
____	____	____	9. Follow package directions to heat the disposable washcloths in microwave. Remove first cloth from bag bath packet or wet washcloth and fold around your finger to make a mitt.	
____	____	____	a. Fold washcloth into thirds.	
____	____	____	b. Straighten washcloth to take out wrinkles.	
____	____	____	c. Fold washcloth over to fit hand.	
____	____	____	d. Tuck loose ends under edge of washcloth on palm.	
____	____	____	10. Cleanse eyes with water only, wiping from inner to outer canthus. Use separate corner of mitt for each eye.	
____	____	____	11. Determine if patient would like soap used on face. Wash face, neck, and ears. Liquid nondetergent cleansing agents are available in some institutions to mix directly into bath water. These products are nondrying and need not be rinsed from the skin. *or* Use first cloth to cleanse face.	

Excellent	Satisfactory	Needs Practice	PROCEDURE 23-2 **Bathing a Patient in Bed** *(Continued)*	Comments
___	___	___	12. Fold bath blanket off arm away from you. Place towel lengthwise under arm. Wash, rinse, and dry the arm using long, firm strokes from the fingers toward the axilla. Wash axilla. Place folded towel and water basin on patient's bed. Soak patient's hand, then wash and rinse. *or* Continue to use disposable bag bath cloths as directed on the package, cleansing parts of the body.	
___	___	___	13. Repeat for hand and arm nearest you.	
___	___	___	14. Apply deodorant or powder according to patient's preferences. Avoid excessive use of powder or inhalation of powder.	
___	___	___	15. Assess bath water temperature and change water if necessary. Side rails should be up.	
___	___	___	16. Place bath towel over chest. Fold bath blanket down to below umbilicus.	
___	___	___	17. Lift bath towel off chest, and bathe chest and abdomen with cloth using long, firm strokes. Give special attention to skin under the breasts and any other skin folds if patient is overweight. Rinse and dry well. Apply a light dusting of bath powder under the breasts or between skin folds.	
___	___	___	18. Help patient don a clean gown.	
___	___	___	19. Expose leg away from you by folding over bath blanket. Be careful to keep perineum covered.	
___	___	___	20. Lift leg, and place bath towel lengthwise under leg. Wash, rinse, and dry leg using long, firm strokes from ankle to thigh.	
___	___	___	21. Wash feet. Rinse and dry well. Pay special attention to space between toes.	
___	___	___	22. Repeat for other leg and foot.	
___	___	___	23. Assess bath water for warmth. Change water if necessary.	
___	___	___	24. Assist patient to side-lying position. Place bath towel along side of back and buttocks to protect linen. Wash, rinse, and dry back and buttocks. Give a backrub with lotion.	
___	___	___	25. Assist patient to supine position. Assess if patient can wash genitals and perineal area independently. If patient needs help, drape with blanket so that only genitals are exposed. Don disposable, clean gloves. Using fresh water and a new cloth, wash, rinse, and dry genitalia and perineum (see text for instructions).	

PROCEDURE 23-2

Bathing a Patient in Bed *(Continued)*

Excellent	Satisfactory	Needs Practice		Comments
____	____	____	26. Complete care according to patient's preference. Apply powder, lotion, cologne. Assist with hair and mouth care. Make bed with clean linen.	
____	____	____	27. Clean equipment and return to appropriate storage area. Perform hand hygiene.	
____	____	____	28. Document procedure.	

Procedure Checklist for Fundamentals of Nursing: Human Health and Function, 7th edition

Name ____________________ Date ____________________

Unit ____________________ Position ____________________

Instructor/Evaluator: ____________________ Position ____________________

PROCEDURE 23-3

Massaging the Back

Goal: Stimulate circulation to the skin; relieve muscle tension; promote comfort and relaxation.

Excellent	Satisfactory	Needs Practice	Step	Comments
____	____	____	1. Identify the patient.	
____	____	____	2. Close door or bed curtains and explain the procedure to the patient and patient's family.	
____	____	____	3. Help patient to side-lying or prone position.	
____	____	____	4. Expose back, shoulders, upper arms, and sacral area. Cover remainder of body with bath blanket.	
____	____	____	5. Perform hand hygiene in warm water. Warm lotion by holding container under running warm water.	
____	____	____	6. Pour small amount of lotion into palms.	
____	____	____	7. Begin massage in sacral area with circular motion. Move hands upward to shoulders, massaging over scapulae in smooth, firm strokes. Without removing hands from skin, continue in smooth strokes to upper arms and down sides of back to iliac crest. Continue for 3 to 5 minutes.	
____	____	____	8. While massaging, assess for broken skin areas and whitish or reddened areas that do not disappear. Do not apply pressure over areas of breakdown or redness.	
____	____	____	9. If additional stimulation is desired, nurse can use pétrissage (kneading) over the shoulders and gluteal area and tapotement (tapping) up and down the spine.	
____	____	____	10. End massage with long, continuous, stroking movements.	
____	____	____	11. Pat excess lubricant dry with towel. Retie patient's gown, and assist to comfortable position.	
____	____	____	12. Perform hand hygiene.	
____	____	____	13. Document procedure.	

Procedure Checklist for Fundamentals of Nursing: Human Health and Function, 7th edition

Name ______________________________ Date ______________

Unit ______________________________ Position ______________

Instructor/Evaluator: ______________________________ Position ______________

PROCEDURE 23-4

Performing Foot and Hand Care

Goal: Maintain skin integrity; provide for patient's comfort and sense of well-being; maintain foot function and ability to ambulate; encourage self-care.

Excellent	Satisfactory	Needs Practice		Comments
____	____	____	1. Perform hand hygiene.	
____	____	____	2. Identify the patient.	
____	____	____	3. Close door or bed curtains and explain the procedure to the patient.	
____	____	____	4. Help patient to chair if possible. Elevate head of bed for bedridden patient.	
____	____	____	5. Fill washbasin with warm water (100° to 104°F [37.7° to 40°C]). Place waterproof pad under basin. Soak patient's hands or feet in basin. Do not soak the feet of a patient with diabetes.	
____	____	____	6. Place call light within reach. Allow hands or feet to soak for 10 to 20 minutes.	
____	____	____	7. Dry the hand or foot that has been soaking. Rewarm water, and allow other extremity to soak while you work on the softened nails.	
____	____	____	8. Gently clean under nails with cuticle stick. If nails are thickened and yellow, patient may have a fungal infection. Wear disposable gloves and eye protection.	
____	____	____	9. Beginning with large toe or thumb, cut nail straight across. Shape nail with file. File rather than cut nails of patients with diabetes or circulatory problems.	
____	____	____	10. Push back cuticle gently with cuticle stick.	
____	____	____	11. Repeat procedure with other nails.	
____	____	____	12. Rinse foot or hand in warm water.	
____	____	____	13. Dry thoroughly with towel, especially between digits.	
____	____	____	14. Apply lotion to hands or feet. Do not apply lotion between the toes of a patient with diabetes.	
____	____	____	15. Help patient to comfortable position.	
____	____	____	16. Remove and dispose of equipment.	
____	____	____	17. Perform hand hygiene.	
____	____	____	18. Document procedure.	

Procedure Checklist for Fundamentals of Nursing: Human Health and Function, 7th edition

Name ______________________ Date ______________________

Unit ______________________ Position ______________________

Instructor/Evaluator: ______________________ Position ______________________

PROCEDURE 23-5

Shampooing Hair of a Bedridden Patient

Goal: Cleanse hair and scalp; promote comfort and self-esteem; apply medication to scalp and hair.

Excellent	Satisfactory	Needs Practice		Comments
____	____	____	1. Perform hand hygiene.	
____	____	____	2. Identify the patient.	
____	____	____	3. Close door or bed curtains and explain the procedure to the patient.	
____	____	____	4. Place waterproof pads under patient's head and shoulders, and remove pillow.	
____	____	____	5. Raise bed to highest position.	
____	____	____	6. Remove any pins from hair. Comb and brush hair thoroughly.	
____	____	____	7. Adjust bed to flat position. Place shampooing basin under head. Place bath towel around shoulders and folded washcloth where neck rests on basin.	
____	____	____	8. Fold bed linens down to waist. Cover upper body with bath blanket.	
____	____	____	9. Place wastebasket with plastic bag under spout of shampoo basin on a chair or table at the bedside.	
____	____	____	10. Using water pitcher, wet hair thoroughly with warm water (approximately 110°F [43.3°C]). Check temperature by placing small amount of water on your wrist.	
____	____	____	11. Before shampooing, use hydrogen peroxide to dissolve matted blood in hair. Peroxide normally feels bubbly and warm. Reassure patient that it will not bleach hair.	
____	____	____	12. Apply small amount of shampoo. Massage scalp with fingertips while making shampoo lather. Start at hairline and work toward neck.	
____	____	____	13. Rinse hair with warm water. Reapply shampoo and repeat massage.	
____	____	____	14. Rinse hair thoroughly with warm water. Clean hair "squeaks" when rubbed between fingers.	
____	____	____	15. Apply small amount of conditioner per patient request. Rinse well.	
____	____	____	16. Squeeze excess moisture from hair. Wrap bath towel around hair. Rub to dry hair and scalp. Use second towel if necessary.	

PROCEDURE 23-5

Shampooing Hair of a Bedridden Patient *(Continued)*

Excellent	Satisfactory	Needs Practice		Comments
____	____	____	17. Remove equipment and wet towels from bed. Place dry towel over patient's shoulders.	
____	____	____	18. Dry hair with hair dryer if necessary. Comb and style.	
____	____	____	19. Help patient to comfortable position.	
____	____	____	20. Dispose of soiled equipment and linen.	
			Variation for Using a Dry Shampoo Cap	
____	____	____	4. Spread towel across patient's chest and place shampoo cap on patient.	
____	____	____	5. Massage scalp so that dry shampoo is evenly distributed.	
____	____	____	6. Wait 1 to 3 minutes for shampoo to fully saturate hair.	
____	____	____	7. Remove and discard shampoo cap.	
____	____	____	8. Use clean towel to dry patient's hair.	
____	____	____	9. Groom and style patient's hair.	
____	____	____	10. Document procedure.	

Procedure Checklist for Fundamentals of Nursing: Human Health and Function, 7th edition

Name ______________________ Date ______________

Unit ______________________ Position ______________

Instructor/Evaluator: ______________________ Position ______________

PROCEDURE 23-6
Providing Oral Care

Excellent	Satisfactory	Needs Practice	**Goal**: Cleanse tooth surfaces to prevent odor and caries; maintain hydrated, intact oral mucosa; promote self-esteem and comfort.	**Comments**
___	___	___	1. Perform hand hygiene.	
___	___	___	2. Identify the patient.	
___	___	___	3. Close door or bed curtains and explain the procedure to the patient.	
___	___	___	4. Help patient to a sitting position. If patient cannot sit, help to a side-lying position.	
___	___	___	5. Place towel under patient's chin.	
___	___	___	6. Moisten toothbrush with water and apply small amount of toothpaste. If patient is anticoagulated or has a clotting disorder, use a very soft toothbrush or a sponge-ended swab to prevent gum bleeding.	
___	___	___	7. Hand toothbrush to patient or don disposable gloves and brush patient's teeth as follows:	
___	___	___	a. Hold toothbrush at a 45-degree angle to the gum line.	
___	___	___	b. Using short, vibrating motions, brush from the gum line to the crown of each tooth. Repeat until outside and inside of teeth and gums are cleaned.	
___	___	___	c. Cleanse biting surfaces by brushing with a back-and-forth stroke.	
___	___	___	d. Brush the tongue lightly. Avoid stimulating the gag reflex.	
___	___	___	8. Have patient rinse mouth thoroughly with water and spit into emesis basin.	
___	___	___	9. Remove emesis basin, set aside, and dry patient's mouth with washcloth.	
___	___	___	10. Floss patient's teeth.	
___	___	___	a. Cut 10-inch piece of dental floss. Wind ends of floss around middle finger of each hand.	
___	___	___	b. Using index fingers to stretch the floss, move the floss up and down around and between lower teeth. Start at the back lower teeth and work around to the other side.	

Excellent	Satisfactory	Needs Practice	PROCEDURE 23-6 **Providing Oral Care** *(Continued)*	Comments
___	___	___	c. Using thumb and index fingers to stretch the floss, repeat procedure on upper teeth.	
___	___	___	d. Have patient rinse mouth thoroughly and spit into emesis basin.	
___	___	___	11. Remove and dispose of supplies. Help patient to comfortable position.	
___	___	___	12. Remove gloves and perform hand hygiene.	
			Variation for the Unconscious Patient	
___	___	___	1. Perform hand hygiene.	
___	___	___	2. Identify the patient.	
___	___	___	3. Close door or bed curtains and explain the procedure to the patient's family.	
___	___	___	4. Place patient in a side-lying position.	
___	___	___	5. Place towel or waterproof pad under patient's chin.	
___	___	___	6. Place emesis basin against patient's mouth or have suction catheter positioned to remove secretions from mouth.	
___	___	___	7. Use padded tongue blade to open teeth gently. Leave in place between the back molars. Never put your fingers in an unconscious patient's mouth.	
___	___	___	8. Brush teeth and gums as directed previously, using toothbrush or soft sponge-ended swab. Cleanse oral cavity using toothette.	
___	___	___	9. Use a small bulb syringe or syringe without needle to rinse oral cavity. Swab or use oral suction to remove pooled secretions.	
___	___	___	10. Apply thin layer of petroleum jelly to lips to prevent drying or cracking.	
___	___	___	11. Document procedure.	

Procedure Checklist for Fundamentals of Nursing: Human Health and Function, 7th edition

Name ______________________ Date ______________

Unit ______________________ Position ______________

Instructor/Evaluator: ______________________ Position ______________

PROCEDURE 23-7
Using a Bedpan

Excellent	Satisfactory	Needs Practice	**Goal:** Provide a means for elimination for patients who are confined to bed or unable to get to the bathroom or bedside commode independently or safely.	Comments
			Placing the Bedpan	
___	___	___	1. Perform hand hygiene. Don clean gloves.	
___	___	___	2. Identify the patient.	
___	___	___	3. Close door or bed curtains and explain the procedure to the patient and patient's family.	
___	___	___	4. Position and lock side rail up on opposite side of bed from which you will work.	
___	___	___	5. Raise bed to height appropriate for nurse.	
___	___	___	6. For patient who can raise buttocks and assist with procedure:	
___	___	___	a. Fold top linen down on your side to expose the patient's hips. (Patient in photographs is exposed for better visualization of procedure.)	
___	___	___	b. Have patient flex knees and lift buttocks. Slide waterproof pad under patient.	
___	___	___	c. Assist patient by placing your hand under sacrum, elbow on mattress, and lifting as a lever. Slide rounded, smooth rim of regular bedpan under patient. If using a fracture pan, slide narrow, flat end under buttocks.	
___	___	___	7. For patient unable to assist by raising buttocks:	
___	___	___	a. Lower head of bed to flat position.	
___	___	___	b. Fold top bed linens down to expose patient minimally.	
___	___	___	c. Help patient to roll to side-lying position.	
___	___	___	d. Place bedpan against buttocks and tucked down against mattress. Hold firmly in place and roll patient onto back as bedpan is positioned under buttocks.	
___	___	___	8. Cover patient with linen. Place call light and toilet paper within reach.	
___	___	___	9. Raise head of bed 45 to 80 degrees unless contraindicated.	
___	___	___	10. Lower bed to lowest position. Place side rails up if indicated.	
___	___	___	11. Perform hand hygiene. Allow patient to be alone.	

Excellent	Satisfactory	Needs Practice	PROCEDURE 23-7 **Using a Bedpan** *(Continued)*	Comments
			Removing the Bedpan	
___	___	___	12. Answer call light promptly.	
___	___	___	13. Place soap, wet washcloth, and towel at bedside.	
___	___	___	14. Raise bed to appropriate working height for nurse.	
___	___	___	15. Fold back top linens to expose patient minimally.	
___	___	___	16. Put on disposable clean gloves.	
___	___	___	17. Assess if patient can wipe perineal area. If not, wipe area with several layers of toilet tissue. If specimen is to be measured or collected, dispose of soiled toilet tissue in separate receptacle, not bedpan. For female patients, wipe from urethra toward anus.	
___	___	___	18. For patient who can raise buttocks and assist with procedure:	
___	___	___	a. Lower head of bed.	
___	___	___	b. Have patient flex knees and lift buttocks. Assist patient by placing one hand under sacrum and supporting bedpan with other hand to prevent spillage. Remove bedpan and place on bedside chair.	
___	___	___	c. Offer soap, warm water, washcloth, and towel for patient to wash hands or perineal area.	
___	___	___	19. For patient unable to assist by raising buttocks:	
___	___	___	a. Lower head of bed to flat position.	
___	___	___	b. Fold top linen down to expose patient minimally.	
___	___	___	c. Help patient to roll off bedpan and onto side. Use one hand to stabilize bedpan during turning to prevent spillage.	
___	___	___	d. Wipe anal area with tissue. Wash perineum with soap and warm water. Pat dry.	
___	___	___	20. Assist patient to comfortable position.	
___	___	___	21. Cover bedpan and remove from bedside. Obtain specimen if required. Empty and clean bedpan, and return it to bedside.	
___	___	___	22. Remove and discard gloves. Perform hand hygiene.	
___	___	___	23. Spray air freshener if necessary to control odor, unless contraindicated (patient with respiratory conditions, allergies).	
___	___	___	24. Document procedure.	

Procedure Checklist for Fundamentals of Nursing: Human Health and Function, 7th edition

Name ______________________ Date ______________________

Unit ______________________ Position ______________________

Instructor/Evaluator: ______________________ Position ______________________

PROCEDURE 23-8

Making an Occupied Bed

Excellent	Satisfactory	Needs Practice	**Goal:** Provide clean linen for patient who is unable to get out of bed; promote comfort.	Comments
___	___	___	1. Perform hand hygiene.	
___	___	___	2. Identify the patient.	
___	___	___	3. Close door or bed curtains and explain the procedure to the patient and patient's family.	
___	___	___	4. Assemble equipment on bedside table or chair. Do not place on another patient's bed.	
___	___	___	5. Lock up side rails on side of bed opposite from where you stack the clean linen.	
___	___	___	6. Raise bed to comfortable working position. Lower side rail on your side of bed.	
___	___	___	7. Loosen all top linen from foot of bed. Remove top linen and bedspread or blanket separately. Without shaking, fold each piece and place over back of chair if it is to be reused. If it is soiled, hold it away from your uniform and place in linen bag.	
___	___	___	8. Leave top sheet on patient or cover patient with a bath blanket; if using bath blanket, remove top sheet from under bath blanket and discard top sheet. (A bath blanket does not appear in photos for better visualization.)	
___	___	___	9. Loosen the bottom sheet on your side. Lower head of bed to flat position. If patient cannot tolerate flat position, lower head of bed as far as patient can tolerate.	
___	___	___	10. Help patient to roll onto side facing away from you. Patient may grasp side rail to assist. Additional personnel may be needed to assist with patient positioning. Adjust pillow under head.	
___	___	___	11. Tightly fanfold soiled linens. Tuck under buttocks, back, and shoulders. Do not fanfold mattress pad unless it is soiled.	
			With Flat Bottom Sheet	
___	___	___	12. Unfold lengthwise so bottom edge is even with end of mattress and vertical center crease is at center of bed.	

Excellent	Satisfactory	Needs Practice	PROCEDURE 23-8 **Making an Occupied Bed** *(Continued)*	Comments
____	____	____	13. Bring sheet's bottom edge over mattress sides and fanfold top of sheet toward center of mattress and place next to patient. Tuck top edge of sheet under mattress. Miter top corner on your side.	
____	____	____	a. Grasp side edge of sheet about 18 inches down from mattress top.	
____	____	____	b. Lay sheet on top of mattress to form a triangular, flat fold.	
____	____	____	c. Tuck sheet hanging loose below mattress under mattress without pulling on the triangular fold.	
____	____	____	d. Pick up triangular fold, and place it over side of the mattress.	
____	____	____	e. Tuck this loose portion of sheet under the mattress.	
____	____	____	14. Tuck remaining portion of sheet under mattress. Proceed to step 16.	
			With Fitted Sheet	
____	____	____	15. Secure the top and bottom elastic edges over the side of the mattress nearest you. Fanfold top of sheet toward center of mattress and place next to patient.	
____	____	____	16. Place draw sheet on bed with center fold at center of bed. Position sheet so it will extend from the patient's back to below the buttocks. Fanfold the top edge and place next to patient. Tuck excess under mattress. Some agencies use a cloth waterproof pad instead of a draw sheet.	
____	____	____	17. Position bottom sheet and draw sheet under soiled sheets.	
____	____	____	18. Lock up side rails on your side and move to other side of bed.	
____	____	____	19. Lower side rail. Help patient to roll over folds of linen onto his or her other side. You may need additional help if patient is unable to move easily. Move pillow under patient's head.	
____	____	____	20. Remove soiled linen by folding into a square or bundle with soiled side turned in. Place in linen bag.	
____	____	____	21. Grasp edge of fanfolded bottom sheet and pull from under the patient.	

PROCEDURE 23-8
Making an Occupied Bed *(Continued)*

Excellent	Satisfactory	Needs Practice		Comments
___	___	___	22. If using flat sheet, tuck top of sheet under top of mattress and miter top corner. Pull bottom sheet tight and tuck excess linen under mattress from top to bottom. If using fitted sheet, secure elastic corners at the head and foot of mattress.	
___	___	___	23. Unfold draw sheet by grasping at center. Pull draw sheet taut and smooth. Tuck excess tightly under mattress. Tuck the middle first, then the top, and finally the bottom.	
___	___	___	24. Help patient to center of bed.	
___	___	___	25. Raise side rail if necessary and move to side of bed where remainder of linen is stored.	
___	___	___	26. Place top sheet over patient with center crease lengthwise at center of bed with seam side up. Unfold sheet from head to toe.	
___	___	___	27. Have patient grasp top edge of clean top sheet. Remove bath blanket or soiled top linen by pulling from beneath clean top sheet. Smooth sheet, with excess falling over bottom edge of mattress.	
___	___	___	28. Discard in linen bag.	
___	___	___	29. Place top sheet on bed with vertical center fold at center of bed. Unfold sheet with seams facing out and top edge even with top of mattress. Smooth sheet, with excess falling over bottom edge of mattress.	
___	___	___	30. Spread blanket or bedspread evenly over bed. Miter the bottom corner, using all layers of linen (sheet, blanket, bedspread). Leave sides untucked. Move to opposite side of bed and repeat.	
___	___	___	31. Standing at bottom of bed, grasp top covers about 10 inches from bottom of mattress. Loosen linen slightly by pulling on top covers or forming a pleat.	
___	___	___	32. Put on clean pillowcases:	
___	___	___	a. Grasp center of pillowcase with one hand on seamed end.	
___	___	___	b. Gather case, turning it inside out over the hand holding it.	
___	___	___	c. With same hand, grasp middle of one end of pillow.	
___	___	___	d. Pull case over pillow with free hand.	
___	___	___	e. Adjust case so corners fit over pillow.	

PROCEDURE 23-8
Making an Occupied Bed *(Continued)*

Excellent	Satisfactory	Needs Practice		Comments
____	____	____	33. Place pillows in center at head of bed.	
____	____	____	34. Ensure that call light is within patient's reach and lower bed.	
____	____	____	35. Arrange the bedside table, night stand, and personal items within easy reach.	
____	____	____	36. Discard soiled linens and wash your hands.	
____	____	____	37. Document procedure.	

Procedure Checklist for Fundamentals of Nursing: Human Health and Function, 7th edition

Name ______________________ Date ______________

Unit ______________________ Position ______________

Instructor/Evaluator: ______________________ Position ______________

PROCEDURE 24-1

Using Body Mechanics to Move Patients

Excellent	Satisfactory	Needs Practice	**Goal:** Prevent injury to the nurse's musculoskeletal system; prevent injury to the patient during transfer.	**Comments**
____	____	____	1. Plan movement before doing it.	
____	____	____	a. Always lock wheels on bed, stretcher, or wheelchair.	
____	____	____	b. Allow patient to assist during move.	
____	____	____	c. Use mechanical aids (e.g., transfer belts, mechanical lifts, slide boards, body mobilizers) or additional personnel to move heavy patients.	
____	____	____	d. When possible, slide, push, or pull patient rather than lift or carry.	
____	____	____	e. Tighten abdominal and gluteal muscles before lifting or moving patient.	
____	____	____	f. Use smooth, rhythmic, coordinated motions.	
____	____	____	g. If another person is assisting, plan your movements before beginning.	
____	____	____	2. Begin all movements with body aligned and balanced.	
____	____	____	a. Face patient to be moved, and plan to pivot your entire body without twisting your back.	
____	____	____	b. Place both feet flat on floor; position your feet and shins alongside the patient's feet and shins; bend knees slightly with one foot slightly in front of the other or one step apart.	
____	____	____	c. Bend knees to lower center of gravity toward patient to be moved.	
____	____	____	3. Grasp transfer belt using an underhand grip or pass your arms under the patient's arms, placing your hands on the patient's upper back. Assist patient to stand.	
____	____	____	4. When possible, elevate adjustable beds to waist level and lower side rails.	
____	____	____	5. Carry objects close to body, and stand as close as possible to work area.	

Procedure Checklist for Fundamentals of Nursing: Human Health and Function, 7th edition

Name ______________________ Date ______________

Unit ______________________ Position ______________

Instructor/Evaluator: ______________________ Position ______________

PROCEDURE 24-2

Positioning a Patient in Bed

Excellent	Satisfactory	Needs Practice	**Goal:** Maintain proper body alignment; maintain skin integrity and prevent deformities of the musculoskeletal system; provide comfort; maintain optimal position for ventilation and lung expansion.	Comments
____	____	____	1. Perform hand hygiene.	
____	____	____	2. Identify the patient as well as any positioning or mobility restrictions.	
____	____	____	3. Close door or bed curtains and explain the procedure to the patient.	
____	____	____	4. Lower head of bed as flat as patient can tolerate. Raise level of bed to comfortable working height.	
____	____	____	5. Remove all pillows from under patient. Leave one at head of bed.	
			Moving a Patient Up in Bed (One Nurse)	
____	____	____	1. Instruct patient to bend legs and put feet flat on bed.	
____	____	____	2. Place your feet in broad stance with one foot in front of the other. Flex your knees and use your thighs.	
____	____	____	3. Place one arm under patient's shoulders and one arm under thighs. Keep head up and back straight. Ask patient to fold the arms across chest, if able. Have patient lift head and place chin on chest.	
____	____	____	4. Rock back and forth on front and back legs to count of three. On third count, have patient push with feet as you lift and assist the patient up in bed.	
____	____	____	5. Elevate head of bed and place pillows under head. Raise side rails and lower bed to lowest level.	
			Moving Helpless Patient Up in Bed (Two Nurses)	
____	____	____	1. One nurse stands on each side of bed with legs positioned for wide base of support and one foot slightly in front of the other.	
____	____	____	2. Each nurse rolls up and grasps edges of turn sheet close to patient's shoulders and buttocks.	
____	____	____	3. Flex knees and hips. Tighten abdominal and gluteal muscles and keep back straight.	

Excellent	Satisfactory	Needs Practice	PROCEDURE 24-2 **Positioning a Patient in Bed** *(Continued)*	Comments
___	___	___	4. Rock back and forth on front and back legs to count of three. On third count, both nurses shift weight to front leg as they simultaneously lift patient toward head of bed.	
___	___	___	5. Elevate head of bed and place pillows under patient's head. Adjust other positioning pillows as necessary. Put up side rails and lower bed to lowest level.	
			Positioning Patient in Side-Lying Position	
___	___	___	1. Elevate and lock side rail on side patient will face when turned.	
___	___	___	2. Using draw sheet, move patient to the edge of the bed, opposite the side on which he or she will be turned.	
___	___	___	3. Place arm that patient will turn toward away from his or her body. Fold other arm across chest.	
___	___	___	4. Flex patient's knee that will not be next to mattress after turn. Have patient reach toward side rail with opposite arm.	
___	___	___	5. Assume a broad stance with knees slightly flexed.	
___	___	___	6. Using draw sheet, gently pull patient over on side.	
___	___	___	7. Align patient properly, then place pillows behind back and under head.	
___	___	___	8. Pull shoulder blade forward and out from under patient. Support patient's upper arm with pillow.	
___	___	___	9. Place pillow lengthwise between patient's legs from thighs to foot.	
___	___	___	10. Cover patient with top linen and blanket. Elevate head of bed. Put up side rails and lower bed to lower level.	
			Logrolling	
___	___	___	1. Obtain assistance. Assess the need for a cervical collar or thoracic braces or jackets to stabilize the spine.	
___	___	___	2. Nurses stand with feet apart, one foot slightly ahead of the other. Flex knees and hips.	
___	___	___	3. Use one pillow to support patient's head during and after turn. Instruct patient to fold arms over chest and keep body stiff. Roll draw sheet toward patient.	
___	___	___	4. Place pillows between patient's legs.	
___	___	___	5. Reach across patient and support head, thorax, trunk, and legs. On count of three, roll patient in one coordinated movement to lateral position.	
___	___	___	6. Support patient in alignment with pillows as described in "Positioning Patient in Side-Lying Position" above. Patients with suspected or known cervical spinal injuries must wear cervical collars.	

Procedure Checklist for Fundamentals of Nursing: Human Health and Function, 7th edition

Name ______________________ Date ______________________

Unit ______________________ Position ______________________

Instructor/Evaluator: ______________________ Position ______________________

PROCEDURE 24-3

Providing Range-of-Motion Exercises

Goal: Maintain joint mobility; improve or maintain muscle strength; prevent muscle atrophy and contractures.

Excellent	Satisfactory	Needs Practice		Comments
___	___	___	1. Perform hand hygiene.	
___	___	___	2. Identify the patient as well as the patient's movement limitations.	
___	___	___	3. Close door or bed curtains and explain the procedure to the patient.	
___	___	___	4. Position patient on back with head of bed as flat as possible. Elevate bed to comfortable working height.	
___	___	___	5. Stand on side of bed where joints are to be exercised. Uncover only the limb to be exercised.	
___	___	___	6. Perform exercises slowly and gently, providing support by holding areas proximal and distal to the joint. Often, this can be done while providing hygiene.	
___	___	___	7. Repeat each exercise five times. Discontinue or decrease ROM if patient complains of discomfort or muscle spasm.	
___	___	___	8. Neck:	
___	___	___	a. Move chin to chest.	
___	___	___	b. Return head to upright position.	
___	___	___	c. Tilt head toward each shoulder.	
___	___	___	d. Move chin toward each shoulder.	
___	___	___	e. Rotate head in circular motion.	
___	___	___	f. Return head to erect position.	
___	___	___	9. Shoulder:	
___	___	___	a. Raise patient's arm from side to above head.	
___	___	___	b. Abduct and rotate shoulder by raising arm above head with palm up.	
___	___	___	c. Adduct shoulder by moving arm across body as far as possible.	
___	___	___	d. Rotate shoulder internally and externally by flexing elbow and moving forearm so the palm touches mattress; then reverse the motion so that back of patient's hand touches mattress.	
___	___	___	e. Move shoulder in a full circle.	

Excellent	Satisfactory	Needs Practice	PROCEDURE 24-3 **Providing Range-of-Motion Exercises** *(Continued)*	Comments
____	____	____	10. Elbow:	
____	____	____	a. Bend elbow so that forearm moves toward shoulder.	
____	____	____	b. Hyperextend elbow as far as possible.	
____	____	____	11. Wrist and hand:	
____	____	____	a. Rotate lower arm and hand so palm is up.	
____	____	____	b. Rotate lower arm and hand so palm is down.	
____	____	____	c. Move hand toward inner aspect of forearm.	
____	____	____	d. Return hand to neutral position.	
____	____	____	e. Bend dorsal surface of hand backward.	
____	____	____	f. Abduct wrist by bending toward thumb.	
____	____	____	g. Adduct wrist by bending toward fifth finger.	
____	____	____	h. Make a fist; extend the fingers.	
____	____	____	i. Spread fingers apart, then together.	
____	____	____	j. Move thumb across hand to base of fifth finger.	
____	____	____	12. Hip and knee:	
____	____	____	a. Lift leg and bend knee toward chest. Return leg to straightened position.	
____	____	____	b. Abduct and adduct leg, moving leg laterally away from body. Return leg to medial position and try to extend it beyond the midpoint.	
____	____	____	c. Internally and externally rotate hip by turning leg inward, then outward.	
____	____	____	d. Take special care to support joints of larger limbs.	
____	____	____	13. Ankle and foot:	
____	____	____	a. Dorsiflex foot by moving it so toes point upward.	
____	____	____	b. Plantarflex by moving foot so toes point downward.	
____	____	____	c. Curl toes down, then extend.	
____	____	____	d. Spread toes apart, then bring together.	
____	____	____	e. Invert by turning sole of foot medially.	
____	____	____	f. Evert by turning sole of foot laterally.	
____	____	____	14. Move to other side of bed and repeat exercises.	
____	____	____	15. Reposition patient comfortably.	
____	____	____	16. Document ROM.	

Procedure Checklist for Fundamentals of Nursing: Human Health and Function, 7th edition

Name ______________________________ Date ______________________

Unit ______________________________ Position ______________________

Instructor/Evaluator: ______________________________ Position ______________________

PROCEDURE 24-4
Assisting With Ambulation

Excellent	Satisfactory	Needs Practice	**Goal:** Promote safe ambulation free from falls or injury; increase muscle strength and joint mobility; prevent complications of immobility; promote self-esteem and independence.	Comments
____	____	____	1. Perform hand hygiene.	
____	____	____	2. Identify the patient.	
____	____	____	3. Close door or bed curtains and explain the procedure and purpose of ambulation to the patient. Decide together how far and where to walk.	
____	____	____	4. Place bed in lowest position.	
____	____	____	5. Assist patient to sitting position on side of bed. Assess for dizziness. Obtain orthostatic vital signs if complaints are present. Allow patient to remain in this position until he or she feels secure.	
____	____	____	6. Help patient with clothing and footwear.	
			One Nurse	
____	____	____	7. Wrap transfer belt around patient's waist (optional according to previous assessment).	
____	____	____	8. Assist patient to standing position and assess patient's balance. Return patient to bed or transfer to chair if he or she is very weak or unsteady. Be sure patient does not grasp your neck for support but places his or her hands around your shoulders or at your waist.	
____	____	____	9. Assess patient position when grasping cane. The handle of the cane should be level with the greater trochanter and should allow approximately 15 degrees of flexion at the elbow.	
____	____	____	10. Position yourself behind patient while supporting him or her by waist or transfer belt.	
____	____	____	11. Take several steps forward with patient. Assess strength and balance. Encourage patient to use good posture and to look ahead, not down at feet.	
____	____	____	12. Ambulate for planned distance or time. If patient becomes weak or dizzy, return patient to bed or assist to chair.	
____	____	____	13. If patient begins to fall, place your feet wide apart with one foot in front. Support patient by pulling his or her weight backward against your body. Lower gently to floor, protecting head.	

Excellent	Satisfactory	Needs Practice	PROCEDURE 24-4 **Assisting With Ambulation** *(Continued)*	Comments
			Two Nurses	
___	___	___	7. Assist patient to sitting position as described.	
___	___	___	8. Assist patient to standing position with one nurse on each side.	
___	___	___	9. One nurse grasps the transfer belt to support the patient. The other nurse may carry and manage equipment.	
___	___	___	10. Walk with patient using slow, even steps. Assess strength and balance. Encourage patient to look forward rather than down at floor.	
			Using a Walker	
___	___	___	7. Assist patient to standing position. Have patient keep one hand on the arm of the chair or bed while she or he assumes an upright posture.	
___	___	___	8. Have patient grasp walker handles. Patient moves walker ahead 6 to 8 inches, placing all four feet of walker on floor. Patient moves forward to walker.	
___	___	___	9. Nurse should walk closely behind and slightly to side of patient. Use a transfer belt if patient is not steady or is at risk for falling.	
___	___	___	10. Repeat above sequence until walk is complete.	

Procedure Checklist for Fundamentals of Nursing: Human Health and Function, 7th edition

Name ______________________ Date ______________________

Unit ______________________ Position ______________________

Instructor/Evaluator: ______________________ Position ______________________

PROCEDURE 24-5

Helping Patients With Crutchwalking

Goal: Increase patient's level of activity after musculoskeletal injury; assist patient to walk safely with crutches using the least amount of energy.

Excellent	Satisfactory	Needs Practice	Procedure	Comments
____	____	____	1. Perform hand hygiene.	
____	____	____	2. Identify the patient.	
____	____	____	3. Close door or bed curtains and explain the procedure to the patient.	
			Four-Point Gait	
____	____	____	4. Patient stands erect, face forward in tripod position. Patient places crutch tips 6 inches in front of feet and 6 inches to side of each foot.	
____	____	____	5. Patient moves right crutch forward 6 inches.	
____	____	____	6. Patient moves left foot forward to level of right crutch.	
____	____	____	7. Patient moves left crutch forward 6 inches.	
____	____	____	8. Patient moves right foot forward to level of left crutch.	
____	____	____	9. Repeat sequence.	
			Three-Point Gait	
____	____	____	4. Beginning in the tripod position, patient moves both crutches and affected leg forward.	
____	____	____	5. Patient moves stronger leg forward.	
____	____	____	6. Repeat sequence.	
			Two-Point Gait	
____	____	____	4. Beginning in the tripod position, patient moves left crutch and right foot forward.	
____	____	____	5. Patient moves right crutch and left foot forward.	
____	____	____	6. Repeat sequence.	
			Swing-To Gait	
____	____	____	4. Patient forms tripod position and moves both crutches forward.	
____	____	____	5. Patient lifts legs and swings to crutches, supporting body weight on crutches.	

PROCEDURE 24-5

Helping Patients With Crutchwalking *(Continued)*

Excellent	Satisfactory	Needs Practice		Comments
			Swing-Through Gait	
___	___	___	4. Patient forms tripod position and moves both crutches forward.	
___	___	___	5. Patient lifts legs and swings through and ahead of crutches, supporting weight on crutches.	
			Climbing Stairs	
___	___	___	4. Use one crutch and the railing. Beginning in tripod position facing stairs, patient transfers body weight to crutches and holds onto the railing.	
___	___	___	5. Patient places unaffected leg on stair.	
___	___	___	6. Patient transfers body weight to unaffected leg.	
___	___	___	7. Patient moves crutches and affected leg to stair.	
___	___	___	8. Repeat sequence to top of stairs.	

Procedure Checklist for Fundamentals of Nursing: Human Health and Function, 7th edition

Name ______________________ Date ______________________

Unit ______________________ Position ______________________

Instructor/Evaluator: ______________________ Position ______________________

PROCEDURE 24-6

Transferring a Patient to a Stretcher

Excellent	Satisfactory	Needs Practice	**Goal:** Transfer a patient without injuring nurse or patient.	**Comments**
___	___	___	1. Perform hand hygiene.	
___	___	___	2. Identify the patient.	
___	___	___	3. Close door or bed curtains and explain the procedure to the patient.	
___	___	___	4. Place stretcher parallel to bed. Raise bed to same level as stretcher. Lower side rails. Lock wheels.	
___	___	___	5. One or two nurses stand on side of bed without stretcher. Two nurses stand on side of bed with stretcher.	
___	___	___	6. Loosen draw sheet on both sides of bed or use turn sheet.	
___	___	___	7. Nurse on side without stretcher helps patient to move toward them onto his or her side. They may use draw sheet to pull patient closer.	
___	___	___	8. Nurse(s) on stretcher side of bed slide transfer board under draw sheet and under patient's buttocks and back.	
___	___	___	9. Place patient's arms across his or her chest. Using draw sheet, slide patient onto transfer board into supine position.	
___	___	___	10. On the count of three, nurse(s) on stretcher side pull the draw sheet toward the stretcher. Nurse on side without transfer board lifts the draw sheet, transferring patient's weight to transfer board and pushing patient onto stretcher.	
___	___	___	11. Roll patient slightly up onto side, and pull transfer board out from under him or her. Lock up side rails on bed side of stretcher and move stretcher away from bed.	
___	___	___	12. Place sheet over patient and lock safety belts across patient's chest and waist. Adjust head of stretcher according to patient limitations.	

Procedure Checklist for Fundamentals of Nursing: Human Health and Function, 7th edition

Name ______________________ Date ______________________

Unit ______________________ Position ______________________

Instructor/Evaluator: ______________________ Position ______________________

PROCEDURE 24-7

Transferring a Patient to a Wheelchair

Excellent	Satisfactory	Needs Practice	**Goal**: Increase mobility status using a wheelchair; prevent complications of immobility; increase independence and promote self-esteem.	**Comments**
____	____	____	1. Perform hand hygiene.	
____	____	____	2. Identify the patient.	
____	____	____	3. Close door or bed curtains and explain the procedure to the patient.	
____	____	____	4. Position wheelchair at 45-degree angle or parallel to bed. Remove footrest and lock brakes.	
____	____	____	5. Lock bed brakes; lower bed to lowest level, and raise head of bed as far as patient can tolerate.	
____	____	____	6. Assist patient to side-lying position, facing the side of bed he or she will sit on. Lower side rail and stand near patient's hips with foot near head of bed in front of and apart from other foot.	
____	____	____	7. Swing patient's legs over side of bed. At the same time, pivot on your back leg to lift patient's trunk and shoulders. Keep back straight; avoid twisting. Allow patient to independently move to a sitting position if he or she can tolerate it. Remain close for support.	
____	____	____	8. Stand in front of patient, and assess for balance and dizziness. Allow patient to dangle legs for a few minutes before continuing.	
____	____	____	9. Help patient to don robe and nonskid footwear.	
____	____	____	10. Apply transfer belt. Grip belt to assist with transfer.	
____	____	____	11. Spread your feet apart and flex your hips and knees.	
____	____	____	12. Have patient slide buttocks to edge of bed until feet touch floor.	
____	____	____	13. Rock back and forth until patient stands on the count of three.	
____	____	____	14. Brace your front knee against patient's weak knee as patient stands.	
____	____	____	15. Pivot on back foot until patient feels wheelchair against back of legs; keep your knee against the patient's knee.	
____	____	____	16. Instruct patient to place hands on chair armrests for support. Flex your knees and hips while assisting patient into chair.	
____	____	____	17. Adjust foot pedal and leg supports.	
____	____	____	18. Assess patient's alignment in chair. Provide call light.	

Procedure Checklist for Fundamentals of Nursing: Human Health and Function, 7th edition

Name ______________________________ Date ______________

Unit ______________________________ Position ______________

Instructor/Evaluator: ______________________________ Position ______________

PROCEDURE 24-8

Procedure for Transferring a Patient From Bed to a Chair Using a Hydraulic Lift

Excellent	Satisfactory	Needs Practice	**Goal:** To safely transfer a patient from a bed to a chair when safe transfer is not possible without using a hydraulic lift.	**Comments**
____	____	____	1. Perform hand hygiene.	
____	____	____	2. Identify the patient.	
____	____	____	3. Close door or bed curtains and explain the procedure to the patient.	
____	____	____	4. Place the fabric sling evenly under the patient.	
____	____	____	5. Position the lift so the frame can be centered over the patient, then attach the fabric sling to the frame. Note manufacturer's instructions for the specifics of how the sling should be attached to the frame.	
____	____	____	6. Have a nurse on each side of the lift. Warn the patient that he or she will be lifted from the bed. Support head or heavy casts as needed. Engage the hydraulic system to raise the patient from the bed.	
____	____	____	7. Carefully wheel the patient in hydraulic lift away from the bed, supporting limbs as needed. Position patient over chair and gently lower to chair using the hydraulic mechanism.	
____	____	____	8. The sling remains in place under the patient and is reattached to the frame when the patient is moved back to bed.	

Procedure Checklist for Fundamentals of Nursing: Human Health and Function, 7th edition

Name ______________________ Date ______________________

Unit ______________________ Position ______________________

Instructor/Evaluator: ______________________ Position ______________________

PROCEDURE 25-1
Monitoring With Pulse Oximetry

Goal: Monitor arterial oxygen saturation (SaO_2) noninvasively; detect clinical hypoxemia promptly; assess patient's tolerance to tapering of oxygen therapy or activity.

Excellent	Satisfactory	Needs Practice		Comments
___	___	___	1. Select appropriate type of sensor. Various sensors are available in sizes for neonates, infants, children, and adults. In addition, there are clip-on, adhesive, and disposable sensors. To select the appropriate sensor, consider the patient's weight, activity level, if infection control is a concern, tape allergies, and anticipated duration of monitoring.	
___	___	___	2. Perform hand hygiene.	
___	___	___	3. Identify the patient.	
___	___	___	4. Close door or bed curtains and explain the procedure to the patient and the family.	
___	___	___	5. Instruct patient to breathe normally.	
___	___	___	6. Select appropriate site to place sensor. Avoid using lower extremities that may have compromised circulation, extremities receiving infusions, or other invasive monitoring. If patient has poor tissue perfusion due to peripheral vascular disease or is receiving vasoconstrictor medications, a nasal sensor or forehead sensor may be considered.	
___	___	___	7. Remove nail polish or acrylic nail from digit to be used.	
___	___	___	8. Attach sensor probe and connect it to the pulse oximeter. Make sure the photosensors are accurately aligned.	
___	___	___	9. Watch for pulse-sensing bar on face of oximeter to fluctuate with each pulsation and reflect pulse strength. Double-check machine pulsations with patient's radial or apical pulse.	
___	___	___	10. If continuous pulse oximetry is desired, set the alarm limits on the monitor to reflect the high and low oxygen saturation and pulse rates. Ensure that the alarms are audible before leaving the patient. Inspect the sensor site every 4 hours for tissue irritation or pressure from the sensor.	
___	___	___	11. Read saturation on monitor and document as appropriate with all relevant information on patient's chart. Report SaO_2 less than 93% to physician.	
___	___	___	12. Document procedure.	

Procedure Checklist for Fundamentals of Nursing: Human Health and Function, 7th edition

Name ______________________ Date ______________________

Unit ______________________ Position ______________________

Instructor/Evaluator: ______________________ Position ______________________

PROCEDURE 25-2

Monitoring Peak Flow

Excellent	Satisfactory	Needs Practice	**Goal**: Measure peak expiratory flow rate (PEFR), which is the point of highest flow during maximal exhalation; better control asthma by quickly detecting subtle changes in airway diameter so that preventive interventions can be instituted; provide objective data to assess respiratory function.	**Comments**
___	___	___	1. Perform hand hygiene.	
___	___	___	2. Identify the patient.	
___	___	___	3. Close door or bed curtains and explain the purpose of peak flow monitoring to the patient and the family.	
___	___	___	4. Place indicator at the base of the numbered scale. Have patient stand up.	
___	___	___	5. Tell the patient to take a deep breath, then place the meter in his or her mouth. The patient should close the lips around the mouthpiece. Remind the patient not to put his or her tongue in the hole.	
___	___	___	6. Tell the patient to exhale as fast and as hard as he or she can, keeping a tight fit around the mouthpiece.	
___	___	___	7. Repeat steps 4 through 6 twice more, and record the highest peak flow obtained in the three attempts.	
___	___	___	8. To determine "personal best" when beginning peak flow monitoring, obtain peak flow measurements in the morning and again in the evening over a 2-week period of good asthma control (feeling good without any asthma symptoms). The patient should take measurements before using bronchodilators.	
___	___	___	9. Healthcare provider will calculate zones based on percentage of personal best (green 80% to 100%, yellow 50% to 80%, red below 50%) and give instructions for what to do when in each zone.	
___	___	___	10. Encourage patient to comply with twice-a-day (morning and evening) peak flow monitoring before bronchodilator therapy and follow healthcare provider's instructions for peak flows in each zone. Follow steps 4 through 7.	
___	___	___	11. Document procedure.	

Procedure Checklist for Fundamentals of Nursing: Human Health and Function, 7th edition

Name ______________________ Date ______________________

Unit ______________________ Position ______________________

Instructor/Evaluator: ______________________ Position ______________________

PROCEDURE 25-3

Teaching Deep Breathing and Coughing

Goal: Facilitate respiratory functioning by increasing lung expansion and preventing alveolar collapse; encourage expectoration of mucus and secretions that accumulate in the airways after general anesthesia and immobility.

Excellent	Satisfactory	Needs Practice		Comments
____	____	____	1. Perform hand hygiene.	
____	____	____	2. Identify the patient.	
____	____	____	3. Close door or bed curtains and explain the procedure to the patient.	
			Deep Breathing	
____	____	____	4. Assist patient to Fowler's or sitting position.	
____	____	____	5. Have patient place hands palm down, with middle fingers touching, along lower border of rib cage.	
____	____	____	6. Ask patient to inhale slowly through the nose, feeling middle fingers separate. Hold breath for 2 or 3 seconds.	
____	____	____	7. Have patient exhale slowly through mouth. Repeat three to five times.	
			Controlled Coughing	
____	____	____	4. If adventitious breath sounds or sputum is present, have patient take a deep breath, hold for 3 seconds, and cough deeply two or three times. Stand to the patient's side to ensure the cough is not directed at you. Patient must cough deeply, not just clear the throat.	
____	____	____	5. If the patient has an abdominal or chest incision that will cause pain during coughing, instruct the patient to hold a pillow firmly over the incision (splinting) when coughing.	
____	____	____	6. Instruct, reinforce, and supervise deep-breathing and coughing exercises every 2 to 3 hours postoperatively.	
____	____	____	7. Document procedure.	

Procedure Checklist for Fundamentals of Nursing: Human Health and Function, 7th edition

Name ________________________ Date ____________

Unit ________________________ Position ____________

Instructor/Evaluator: ________________________ Position ____________

PROCEDURE 25-4

Promoting Breathing With the Incentive Spirometer

Excellent	Satisfactory	Needs Practice	**Goal:** Provides incentives via visual clues to the patient regarding effective deep breathing; improves pulmonary ventilation and oxygenation, loosens respiratory secretions, and prevents or treats atelectasis by expanding collapsed alveoli.	**Comments**
____	____	____	1. Perform hand hygiene.	
____	____	____	2. Identify the patient.	
____	____	____	3. Close door or bed curtains and explain the procedure to the patient.	
____	____	____	4. Assist patient to high Fowler's or sitting position.	
____	____	____	5. Determine the volume to set incentive spirometry goal based on calculated lung volumes. You may use chart or have respiratory therapy calculated. Set volume indicator. Explain goal to patient.	
____	____	____	6. Instruct patient in procedure:	
____	____	____	a. Seal lips tightly around mouthpiece.	
____	____	____	b. Inhale slowly and deeply through mouth. Hold breath for 2 or 3 seconds.	
____	____	____	c. Have patient observe his or her progress by watching the balls elevate or lights go on, depending on type of equipment used.	
____	____	____	d. Exhale slowly around mouthpiece and breathe normally for several breaths.	
____	____	____	7. Repeat procedure 5 to 10 times every 1 to 2 hours, per physician's orders.	
____	____	____	8. Document procedure.	

Procedure Checklist for Fundamentals of Nursing: Human Health and Function, 7th edition

Name ______________________ Date ______________________

Unit ______________________ Position ______________________

Instructor/Evaluator: ______________________ Position ______________________

PROCEDURE 25-5

Administering Oxygen by Nasal Cannula or Mask

Goal: Deliver low to moderate levels of oxygen to relieve hypoxia.

Excellent	Satisfactory	Needs Practice	Step	Comments
____	____	____	1. Review for physician's order for oxygen to ensure that it includes method of delivery, flow rate, titration orders.	
____	____	____	2. Perform hand hygiene.	
____	____	____	3. Identify the patient.	
____	____	____	4. Close door or bed curtains and explain the procedure to the patient. Proceed with the six rights of medication administration. Explain that oxygen will ease dyspnea or discomfort, and inform patient concerning safety precautions associated with oxygen use. If the patient is using the cannula, encourage him or her to breathe through the nose.	
____	____	____	5. Assist patient to semi- or high Fowler's position, if tolerated.	
____	____	____	6. Insert flow meter into wall outlet. Attach oxygen tubing to nozzle on flow meter. If using a high O_2 flow, attach humidifier. Attach oxygen tubing to humidifier.	
____	____	____	7. Turn on the oxygen at the prescribed rate. Check that oxygen is flowing through tubing.	
____	____	____	8. Cannula:	
____	____	____	a. Hold nasal cannula in proper position with prongs curving downward.	
____	____	____	b. Place cannula prongs into nares.	
____	____	____	c. Wrap tubing over and behind ears.	
____	____	____	d. Adjust plastic slide under chin until cannula fits snugly.	
____	____	____	e. Place gauze at ear beneath tubing as necessary.	
____	____	____	f. If prongs dislodge from nares, replace promptly.	
____	____	____	9. Mask:	
____	____	____	a. Place mask on face, applying from the nose and over the chin.	
____	____	____	b. Adjust the metal rim over the nose and contour the mask to the face.	
____	____	____	c. Adjust elastic band around head so mask fits snugly.	

PROCEDURE 25-5

Administering Oxygen by Nasal Cannula or Mask *(Continued)*

Excellent	Satisfactory	Needs Practice		Comments
____	____	____	10. Assess for proper functioning of equipment and observe patient's initial response to therapy.	
____	____	____	11. Monitor continuous therapy by assessing for pressure areas on the skin and nares every 2 hours and rechecking flow rate every 4 to 8 hours.	
____	____	____	12. Document procedure.	

Procedure Checklist for Fundamentals of Nursing: Human Health and Function, 7th edition

Name ______________________ Date ______________________

Unit ______________________ Position ______________________

Instructor/Evaluator: ______________________ Position ______________________

PROCEDURE 25-6
Providing Tracheostomy Care

Excellent	Satisfactory	Needs Practice	**Goal:** Maintain airway patency by removing mucus and encrusted secretions; promote cleanliness and prevent infection and skin breakdown at stoma site.	Comments
____	____	____	1. Verify the physician order.	
____	____	____	2. Perform hand hygiene and don gloves.	
____	____	____	3. Identify the patient.	
____	____	____	4. Close door or bed curtains and explain the procedure to the patient. Place the patient in semi- to high Fowler's position.	
____	____	____	5. Suction tracheostomy tube. Before discarding gloves, remove soiled tracheostomy dressing and discard with catheter inside glove. (*Note:* Follow Procedure 25-7, Suctioning Secretions From Airways. When suctioning through a tracheostomy tube, insert catheter about 10 to 12 cm [in an adult].)	
____	____	____	6. Replace oxygen or humidification source and encourage patient to deep breathe as you prepare sterile supplies. Do not snap in place.	
____	____	____	7. Open sterile tracheostomy kit. Pour normal saline into one basin, hydrogen peroxide into the second. Don sterile gloves. Open several sterile cotton-tipped applicators and one sterile precut tracheostomy dressing, and place on sterile field. If kit does not contain tracheostomy ties, cut two 15-inch pieces of twill tape and set aside.	
____	____	____	8. Remove oxygen source. The hand that touches the oxygen source is no longer sterile. (*Note:* For tracheostomy tube with inner cannula, complete steps 7 to 25. For tracheostomy tube without inner cannula or plugged with a button, complete steps 15 to 26.)	
____	____	____	9. Unlock inner cannula by turning counterclockwise. Remove inner cannula.	
____	____	____	10. Place inner cannula in basin with hydrogen peroxide.	
____	____	____	11. Replace oxygen source over or near outer cannula.	
____	____	____	12. Clean lumen and sides of inner cannula using pipe cleaners or sterile brush.	
____	____	____	13. Rinse inner cannula thoroughly by agitating in normal saline for several seconds.	

Excellent	Satisfactory	Needs Practice	PROCEDURE 25-6 **Providing Tracheostomy Care** *(Continued)*	Comments
___	___	___	14. Remove oxygen source and replace inner cannula into outer cannula, then "lock" by turning clockwise until the two blue dots align. Replace oxygen or humidity source.	
___	___	___	15. Remove tracheostomy dressing from under faceplate.	
___	___	___	16. Clean stoma under faceplate with circular motion using hydrogen peroxide–soaked cotton applicators. Clean dried secretions from all exposed outer cannula surfaces.	
___	___	___	17. Remove foaming secretions using normal saline-soaked, cotton-tipped applicators.	
___	___	___	18. Pat moist surfaces dry with 4″ × 4″ gauze.	
___	___	___	19. Place dry, sterile, precut tracheostomy dressing around tracheostomy stoma and under faceplate. Do not use cut 4″ × 4″ gauze.	
___	___	___	20. If tracheostomy ties are to be changed, have an assistant don a sterile glove and hold the tracheostomy tube in place.	
			For Tracheostomy Ties, Follow Steps 21 Through 25	
___	___	___	21. Cut a ½-inch slit approximately 1 inch from one end of both clean tracheostomy ties. This is easily done by folding back on itself 1 inch of the tie and cutting a small slit in the middle.	
___	___	___	22. Remove and discard soiled tracheostomy ties.	
___	___	___	23. Thread end of tie through cut slit in tie. Pull tight.	
___	___	___	24. Repeat step 22 with the second tie.	
___	___	___	25. Bring both ties together at one side of the patient's neck. Assess that ties are only tight enough to allow one finger between tie and neck. Use two square knots to secure the ties. Trim excess tie length. (*Note:* Assess tautness of tracheostomy ties frequently in patients whose neck may swell from trauma or surgery.)	
			For Tracheostomy Collar, Follow Steps 26 Through 28	
___	___	___	26. While an assisting nurse holds the faceplate, gently pull the Velcro tab and remove the collar on one side. Insert the new collar into the opening on the faceplate and secure the Velcro tab.	
___	___	___	27. Hold faceplate in place as the assisting nurse repeats step on the second side.	
___	___	___	28. Remove the old collar and ensure that the new collar is securely in place.	

Excellent	Satisfactory	Needs Practice	PROCEDURE 25-6 **Providing Tracheostomy Care** *(Continued)*	Comments
____	____	____	29. Remove gloves and discard disposable equipment. Label with date and time, and store reusable supplies.	
____	____	____	30. Assist patient to comfortable position and offer oral hygiene.	
____	____	____	31. Perform hand hygiene.	
____	____	____	32. Document procedure.	

Procedure Checklist for Fundamentals of Nursing: Human Health and Function, 7th edition

Name ______________________ Date ______________________

Unit ______________________ Position ______________________

Instructor/Evaluator: ______________________ Position ______________________

PROCEDURE 25-7
Suctioning Secretions From Airways

Excellent	Satisfactory	Needs Practice	**Goal:** Remove excess mucous secretions to maintain patent airway; collect sputum or secretions for diagnostic testing.	Comments
____	____	____	1. Verify the physician order and identify the patient.	
____	____	____	2. Perform hand hygiene.	
____	____	____	3. Identify the patient.	
____	____	____	4. Close door or bed curtains and explain the procedure to the patient and the family.	
____	____	____	5. a. Position the conscious patient with an intact gag reflex in a semi-Fowler's position.	
____	____	____	b. Position the unconscious patient in a side-lying position facing you.	
____	____	____	6. Turn on suction device and adjust pressure: infants and children, 50 to 75 mm Hg; adults, 100 to 120 mm Hg.	
			7. Open and prepare sterile suction catheter kit:	
____	____	____	a. Unfold sterile cup, touching only the outside. Place on bedside table.	
____	____	____	b. Pour sterile saline into cup.	
____	____	____	8. Preoxygenate patient with 100% oxygen; hyperinflate with manual resuscitation bag.	
____	____	____	9. Don sterile gloves. If kit provides only one glove, place on dominant hand.	
____	____	____	10. Pick up catheter with dominant hand. Pick up connecting tubing with nondominant hand. The nondominant hand is now considered clean rather than sterile. Attach catheter to tubing without contaminating sterile hand.	
____	____	____	11. Place catheter end into cup of saline. Test functioning of equipment by applying thumb from nondominant hand over open port to create suction.	
____	____	____	12. Insert catheter into trachea through nostril, nasal trumpet, or artificial airway during inspiration and without suction.	
____	____	____	13. Advance catheter until you feel resistance. Retract catheter 1 cm before applying suction. (*Note:* Patient usually will cough when catheter enters trachea.)	

PROCEDURE 25-7

Suctioning Secretions From Airways *(Continued)*

Excellent	Satisfactory	Needs Practice		Comments
___	___	___	14. Apply suction by placing thumb of nondominant hand over open port, then rotate the catheter with your dominant hand as you withdraw the catheter. This should take 5 to 10 seconds.	
___	___	___	15. Hyperoxygenate and hyperinflate using manual resuscitation bag for a full minute between subsequent suction passes. Encourage deep breathing.	
___	___	___	16. Rinse catheter thoroughly with saline.	
___	___	___	17. Repeat steps 11 to 15 until airway is clear, limiting each suctioning to three passes.	
___	___	___	18. Without applying suction, insert the catheter gently along one side of the mouth. Advance to the oropharynx.	
___	___	___	19. Apply suction for 5 to 10 seconds as you rotate and withdraw catheter.	
___	___	___	20. Allow 1 to 2 minutes between passes for the patient to ventilate. Encourage deep breathing. Replace oxygen if applicable.	
___	___	___	21. Repeat steps 17 and 18 as necessary to clear oropharynx.	
___	___	___	22. Rinse catheter and tubing by suctioning saline through.	
___	___	___	23. Remove gloves by holding catheter with dominant hand and pulling glove off inside out. Catheter will remain coiled inside the glove. Pull other glove off inside out. Dispose of in trash receptacle.	
___	___	___	24. Turn off suction device. Assist patient to comfortable position. Offer assistance with oral and nasal hygiene. Replace oxygen device if used.	
___	___	___	25. Perform hand hygiene.	
___	___	___	26. Ensure that sterile suction kit is available at head of bed.	
___	___	___	27. Document procedure.	

Procedure Checklist for Fundamentals of Nursing: Human Health and Function, 7th edition

Name ______________________ Date ______________________

Unit ______________________ Position ______________________

Instructor/Evaluator: ______________________ Position ______________________

PROCEDURE 25-8

Monitoring a Patient With a Chest Drainage System

Excellent	Satisfactory	Needs Practice	**Goal:** Monitor respiratory status of a patient with a chest tube; ensure chest drainage system is functioning adequately to promote lung expansion.	Comments
____	____	____	1. Confirm physician's order including amount of suction.	
____	____	____	2. Perform hand hygiene.	
____	____	____	3. Identify the patient.	
____	____	____	4. Close door or bed curtains and explain the procedure to the patient.	
____	____	____	5. Assist patient to semi- or high Fowler's position.	
____	____	____	6. Assess insertion site of chest tube. Note and document amount and color of drainage on dressing around insertion site. Feel insertion site for crepitus—air leaking into the subcutaneous tissue. Document any crepitus found. Reinforce insertion dressing as needed.	
____	____	____	7. Assess status of chest tubing. Be sure tubing remains at the level of the patient and no dependent loops are present. Assess that there are no visible clots in the tubing. You may gently "milk" (compress tubing with fingers) the clots to encourage movement into the drainage system, but you never want to strip chest tubing.	
____	____	____	8. Assess the drainage collection chamber. Be sure to keep chest drainage system upright. Assess for amount, color, and character of drainage. Mark the collection chamber to accurately reflect the amount of drainage accumulated during your shift. Note any significant increase in the amount of drainage.	
____	____	____	9. Assess suction chamber. Make sure the water level in the suction chamber is at the prescribed amount of suction and that it is connected to the wall suction that is turned on to continuous suction. Usually, the suction is set at 10 to 20 mm Hg.	
____	____	____	10. Assess the system for any air leaks. Check all external connections (i.e., the chest tube's connection to the drainage system, the suction tubing's connection to the drainage system). Examine the water seal chamber as the patient breathes normally and as he or she coughs.	

PROCEDURE 25-8

Monitoring a Patient With a Chest Drainage System *(Continued)*

Excellent	Satisfactory	Needs Practice		Comments
____	____	____	11. Encourage the patient to cough, deep breathe, and use an incentive spirometer frequently. Provide analgesics as necessary.	
____	____	____	12. Clamping chest tubes is no longer recommended.	
____	____	____	13. If the chest tube becomes expelled, do not leave the patient. Cover the opening where the chest tube had been inserted with the sterile 4″ × 4″ gauze, and keep direct pressure on the site. Send a colleague to call the physician immediately.	
____	____	____	14. Document chest tube drainage, chest tube patency, air leak, amount of suction, pain level, dressing status, and respiratory status.	

Procedure Checklist for Fundamentals of Nursing: Human Health and Function, 7th edition

Name ______________________ Date ______________________

Unit ______________________ Position ______________________

Instructor/Evaluator: ______________________ Position ______________________

PROCEDURE 25-9

Managing an Obstructed Airway (Heimlich Maneuver)

Excellent	Satisfactory	Needs Practice	**Goal:** Remove a foreign body from obstructing the airway to prevent anoxia and cardiopulmonary arrest.	Comments
			Conscious Child or Adult (Heimlich Maneuver)	
___	___	___	1. The patient will be standing or sitting. Stand behind the patient. Wrap your arms around patient's waist. Make a fist with one hand. Place thumb side of fist against patient's abdomen, above the navel but below the xiphoid process.	
___	___	___	2. Grasp fist with other hand. Press fist into abdomen with a quick upward thrust.	
___	___	___	3. Repeat distinct separate thrusts until the patient expels the foreign body or becomes unconscious.	
			Unconscious Patient (Heimlich Maneuver, Abdominal Thrust)	
___	___	___	1. Patient will be lying on the ground. Turn patient on back and call for help. Activate emergency response system.	
			2. Finger sweep:	
___	___	___	a. Use tongue–jaw lift to open mouth.	
___	___	___	b. Insert index finger inside cheek and sweep to base of tongue if an object is visible. Use a hooking motion, if possible, to dislodge and remove the foreign body. (*Note:* Avoid finger sweeps in infants and children because you can easily push the foreign body further into the airway. Remove only if clearly visible and easy to reach.)	
___	___	___	c. If there is no effective breathing, attempt to provide two rescue breaths. If unsuccessful, reposition and try to ventilate again.	
___	___	___	3. Straddle patient's thighs or kneel to the side of thighs. Place heel of one hand on epigastric area, midline above the navel but below the xiphoid process. Place second hand on top of first hand.	
___	___	___	4. Press heel of hand into abdomen with a quick upward thrust. (*Note:* Be careful to thrust in the midline to prevent injury to the liver or spleen.)	
___	___	___	5. Repeat abdominal thrusts five times. If airway is still obstructed, attempt to ventilate using mouth-to-mouth respiration and head tilt/chin lift. Repeat steps 5 through 8 until successful.	

Excellent	Satisfactory	Needs Practice	PROCEDURE 25-9 **Managing an Obstructed Airway (Heimlich Maneuver)** *(Continued)*	Comments
			Children Younger Than 1 Year of Age (Back Blows and Chest Thrusts)	
____	____	____	1. Straddle infant over your arm with head lower than trunk.	
____	____	____	2. Support head by holding jaw firmly in your hand.	
____	____	____	3. Rest your forearm on your thigh and deliver five back blows with the heel of your hand between the infant's scapula.	
____	____	____	4. Place free hand on infant's back and support neck while turning to supine position.	
____	____	____	5. Place two fingers over sternum in same location as for external chest compression (one fingerwidth below nipple line).	
____	____	____	6. Administer five chest thrusts.	
____	____	____	7. Repeat steps 1 through 6 until airway is not obstructed.	
			Children Older Than 1 Year of Age	
____	____	____	1. Perform Heimlich maneuver with child standing, sitting, or lying as for adult, but more gently.	
____	____	____	2. You may need to kneel behind child or have child stand on a table.	
____	____	____	3. Prevent foreign body airway obstruction in infants and children by teaching parents or caregivers to do the following:	
____	____	____	a. Restrict children from walking, running, or playing with food or foreign objects in their mouths.	
____	____	____	b. Keep small objects (e.g., marbles, beads, beans, thumb tacks) away from children younger than 3 years of age.	
____	____	____	c. Avoid feeding popcorn and peanuts to children younger than 3 years of age, and cut other foods into small pieces.	
____	____	____	4. Instruct parents and caregivers in the management of foreign body airway obstruction.	
			Pregnant Women or Very Obese Adults (Chest Thrusts)	
____	____	____	1. Stand behind patient.	
____	____	____	2. Bring your arms under patient's armpits and around chest.	
____	____	____	3. Make a fist and place thumb side against middle of sternum.	
____	____	____	4. Grasp fist with other hand and deliver a quick backward thrust.	
____	____	____	5. Repeat thrusts until airway is cleared.	
____	____	____	6. Chest thrusts may be performed with patient supine and hands positioned with heel over lower half of sternum (as for cardiac compression). Administer separate downward thrusts until airway is clear.	
____	____	____	7. Document procedure.	

Procedure Checklist for Fundamentals of Nursing: Human Health and Function, 7th edition

Name ______________________ Date ______________________

Unit ______________________ Position ______________________

Instructor/Evaluator: ______________________ Position ______________________

PROCEDURE 26-1

Applying Antiembolic Stockings

Goal: Promote supplementing the action of muscle contraction by venous return from the legs; prevent DVT in the immobile or postoperative patient.

Excellent	Satisfactory	Needs Practice		Comments
____	____	____	1. Perform hand hygiene.	
____	____	____	2. Identify the patient.	
____	____	____	3. Close door or bed curtains and explain procedure to the patient.	
____	____	____	4. Position patient in supine position for a half hour before applying stockings.	
____	____	____	5. Measure for proper fit before first application. Measure length (heel to groin) and width (calf and thigh) and compare to manufacturer's printed material to ensure proper fit.	
____	____	____	6. Make sure legs are dry or apply a light dusting of powder.	
____	____	____	7. Turn the stocking inside out, tucking the foot inside.	
____	____	____	8. Ease foot section over the patient's toe and heel, adjusting as necessary for proper smooth fit.	
____	____	____	9. Gently pull the stocking over the leg, removing all wrinkles.	
____	____	____	10. Assess toes for circulation and warmth. Check area at top of stocking for binding.	
____	____	____	11. Antiembolic stockings should be removed at least twice daily.	

Procedure Checklist for Fundamentals of Nursing: Human Health and Function, 7th edition

Name ______________________ Date ______________________

Unit ______________________ Position ______________________

Instructor/Evaluator: ______________________ Position ______________________

PROCEDURE 26-2

Applying a Sequential Compression Device

Excellent	Satisfactory	Needs Practice	**Goal:** Promote venous return from legs to decrease the risk of DVT and pulmonary embolism in patients with reduced mobility.	Comments
____	____	____	1. Perform hand hygiene.	
____	____	____	2. Identify the patient.	
____	____	____	3. Close door or bed curtains and explain procedure to the patient.	
____	____	____	4. Measure leg to ensure proper sleeve sizing. (*Note:* Knee length—one size fits all; thigh length—measure length of leg from ankle to popliteal fossa.) Measure circumference of thigh at the gluteal fold. Use the correct sleeve size, as follows: extra small (circumference, 22 inches; length, 16 inches), regular (circumference, 29 inches; length, 16 inches), extra large (circumference, 35 inches; length, 16 inches).	
____	____	____	5. Apply antiembolism stockings. Ensure that there are no wrinkles or folds (see Procedure 26-1). (*Note:* Stockinette or Ace wraps are recommended options if patient cannot be fitted with antiembolism stockings.)	
____	____	____	6. Place patient in supine position.	
____	____	____	7. Place a plastic sleeve under each leg so that the opening is at the knee. If only one sleeve is required, leave the other sleeve in package and connect to control unit.	
____	____	____	8. Fold the outer section of the sleeve over the inner portion and secure with Velcro tabs. Check sleeve fit. Two fingers should fit between the sleeve and leg.	
____	____	____	9. Connect tubing to control unit. The premarked arrows on the tubing from the sleeve and from the controller must be aligned to make adequate connection. Turn machine on.	
____	____	____	10. Adjust control unit settings as necessary. Unit control is preset with sleeve cooling in "off" position and audible alarm in "on" position. Sleeve cooling should be in "on" position at all times except during surgery. Ankle pressure should be set at 35 to 55 mm Hg.	
____	____	____	11. Recheck control unit settings whenever unit has been turned off.	

Excellent	Satisfactory	Needs Practice	PROCEDURE 26-2 **Applying a Sequential Compression Device** *(Continued)*	Comments
___	___	___	12. Respond to and promptly correct all "fault" indicator alarms. (*Note:* The control unit will sense and indicate four pressure "fault" conditions: (a) pressure failed to drop to zero during the cycle; (b) the ankle pressure failed to reach 20 mm Hg for five consecutive cycles; (c) the ankle pressure exceeded 90 mm Hg; (d) an internal diagnostics error has occurred.)	
___	___	___	13. Document time and date of application. If SCD is applied to only one leg, document reason.	
___	___	___	14. Assess and document skin integrity every 8 hours.	
___	___	___	15. Remove sleeves and notify physician if patient experiences tingling, numbness, or leg pain.	

Procedure Checklist for Fundamentals of Nursing: Human Health and Function, 7th edition

Name ______________________ Date ______________________

Unit ______________________ Position ______________________

Instructor/Evaluator: ______________________ Position ______________________

PROCEDURE 28-1

Measuring Blood Glucose by Skin Puncture

Excellent	Satisfactory	Needs Practice	**Goal**: Monitor blood glucose levels for patients who are at risk for hypoglycemia or hyperglycemia; monitor the effectiveness of insulin administration.	**Comments**
____	____	____	1. Review the provider's orders to determine the type and frequency of glucose monitoring. (*Note:* The procedure should be performed before meals because carbohydrate ingestion alters blood glucose levels.)	
____	____	____	2. Perform hand hygiene.	
____	____	____	3. Identify the patient.	
____	____	____	4. Close door or bed curtains and explain the procedure to the patient.	
____	____	____	5. Have the patient wash hands with soap and warm water.	
____	____	____	6. Position patient comfortably.	
____	____	____	7. Remove the test strip from the container and handle according to the manufacturer's instructions.	
____	____	____	8. Place the test strip with test pad up on a dry surface.	
____	____	____	9. Don gloves.	
____	____	____	10. Choose the finger to be punctured, massage gently, and hold in a dependent position.	
____	____	____	11. Wipe the puncture site with alcohol. Allow the site to dry completely.	
____	____	____	12. Remove the cover of the lancet or autolet. Place the autolet against the side of the finger and push the release button. If using a lancet, hold it perpendicular to the site and pierce the site quickly.	
____	____	____	13. Squeeze the finger gently or milk the skin toward the puncture site to obtain a large drop of blood. Hold the test strip next to the drop of blood and allow the blood to cover the test pad completely. Do not smear the blood. In some meters, bring the finger to the test site on the meter and allow blood to drop and wick along the test strip, covering the test strip area.	
____	____	____	14. Start the timing (usually less than 60 seconds) using the glucose meter, or use a watch if the meter is not available.	

PROCEDURE 28-1

Measuring Blood Glucose by Skin Puncture *(Continued)*

Excellent	Satisfactory	Needs Practice		Comments
___	___	___	15. Insert the test strip into the glucose meter. After the recommended period, read the results. For meters on which blood is placed directly, read the results at the designated time. If a glucose meter is not available, compare the color of the test pad with the color strip on the side of the reagent strip container.	
___	___	___	16. Turn off the glucose meter. Dispose of used equipment in the appropriate manner.	
___	___	___	17. Share test results with patient and record obtained values in the patient's chart.	
___	___	___	18. Document procedure.	

Procedure Checklist for Fundamentals of Nursing: Human Health and Function, 7th edition

Name ______________________ Date ______________________

Unit ______________________ Position ______________________

Instructor/Evaluator: ______________________ Position ______________________

PROCEDURE 28-2
Assisting an Adult With Feeding

Excellent	Satisfactory	Needs Practice	**Goal:** Maintain nutritional status; provide a time for socialization.	**Comments**
___	___	___	1. Review physician's orders for type of diet.	
___	___	___	2. Identify the patient.	
___	___	___	3. Close door or bed curtains and explain the procedure to the patient and patient's family.	
___	___	___	4. Prepare patient's environment for meal:	
___	___	___	a. Remove urinals, bedpans, dressings, trash.	
___	___	___	b. Ventilate or aerate room for unpleasant odors.	
___	___	___	c. Clean overbed table.	
___	___	___	5. Prepare patient for meal:	
___	___	___	a. Help client urinate or defecate.	
___	___	___	b. Help patient wash face and hands.	
___	___	___	c. Assist with oral hygiene.	
___	___	___	d. Help patient apply dentures, glasses, or special appliances.	
___	___	___	e. Assist patient to upright position in bed or chair.	
___	___	___	6. Perform hand hygiene.	
___	___	___	7. Check patient's tray against diet order and with patient's identification.	
___	___	___	8. Place tray on overbed table and move in front of patient.	
___	___	___	9. Place a napkin or towel under patient's chin, and cover clothing. Prepare tray. Open cartons, remove lids, season food, cut food into bite-size pieces.	
___	___	___	10. If patient can feed self, you may leave at this point, assuring that call light is within reach. Return after 10 to 15 minutes to determine whether patient is tolerating diet. Do not leave patients with overly hot liquids or food unless they are fully independent with feeding.	
___	___	___	11. Assist patients who cannot feed themselves. If patient can sit in a chair but needs help to eat, sit in chair facing patient. If patient must remain in bed, sit in chair (depending on chair height) or stand to feed patient.	
___	___	___	12. Allow patient to choose the order he or she would like to eat. If patient is visually impaired, identify the food on the tray.	

PROCEDURE 28-2

Assisting an Adult With Feeding *(Continued)*

Excellent	Satisfactory	Needs Practice		Comments
____	____	____	13. Warn patient if food is hot or cold. Allow enough time between bites for adequate chewing and swallowing.	
____	____	____	14. Offer liquids as requested or between bites. Use a straw or special drinking cup if available.	
____	____	____	15. Provide conversation during meal. Choose topic of interest to patient. Reorient to current events, or use meal as an opportunity to educate on nutrition or discharge plans. However, do not talk to patients who are relearning swallowing techniques; they need to concentrate.	
____	____	____	16. Remove and dispose of tray. Help patient wash hands and face and perform oral hygiene after meal.	
____	____	____	17. Assist patient to comfortable position, and allow rest period. (*Note:* If client is at risk for aspiration, leave head of bed elevated for 30 minutes after eating.)	
____	____	____	18. Perform hand hygiene.	
____	____	____	19. Document fluids and amount of meal consumed, if ordered.	

Procedure Checklist for Fundamentals of Nursing: Human Health and Function, 7th edition

Name ______________________ Date ______________________

Unit ______________________ Position ______________________

Instructor/Evaluator: ______________________ Position ______________________

PROCEDURE 28-3

Administering Specialized Nutritional Support Via Small-Bore Nasogastric, Gastrostomy, or Jejunostomy Tube

Goal: Provide enteral nutrition for patients who cannot swallow or who have an esophageal obstruction; provide nutrition to comatose or semiconscious patients; provide additional nutrients for patients who cannot orally consume adequate calories.

Excellent	Satisfactory	Needs Practice	Step	Comments
___	___	___	1. Review chart for food allergies and provider's order for type, amount, rate, route, and frequency of feeding.	
___	___	___	2. Perform hand hygiene and don gloves.	
___	___	___	3. Identify the patient.	
___	___	___	4. Close door or bed curtains and explain the procedure to the patient.	
___	___	___	5. Help patient to Fowler's position by elevating head of bed at least 30 to 45 degrees or assisting to a chair. If an upright position is contraindicated, help patient to a right side-lying position with head elevated 30 degrees.	
___	___	___	6. Confirm placement of tube. Attach a 60-mL irrigation (feeding) syringe to tube and inject 10 to 20 mL of air while auscultating with the stethoscope.	
___	___	___	7. Check GRVs.	
___	___	___	a. If GRVs are requested, note amount aspirated in documentation. Notify provider if GRV exceeds 400 to 500 mL.	
___	___	___	b. Replace all gastric contents after residual check.	
___	___	___	8. Prepare correct amount and strength of formula. Formula should be room temperature.	
___	___	___	9. Select steps 10a through 16a below for bolus or intermittent feeding or steps 10b through 18b below for continuous feeding.	
			Bolus or Intermittent Feeding	
___	___	___	10a. Remove plunger from irrigation syringe. Clamp gastric tubing and attach syringe or feeding bag. If using a feeding bag, prime the tubing and attach feeding bag and tubing to the patient's feeding tube.	

Excellent	Satisfactory	Needs Practice	PROCEDURE 28-3 **Administering Specialized Nutritional Support Via Small-Bore Nasogastric, Gastrostomy, or Jejunostomy Tube** *(Continued)*	Comments
___	___	___	11a. Fill syringe or feeding bag with formula. Allow feeding to flow in slowly (10 to 15 minutes). If using syringe, raise or lower syringe to adjust flow rate by gravity. Refill syringe as needed without disconnecting, avoiding air-spaces in tubing. If a feeding bag is used, hang bag on IV pole, and adjust flow rate with clamp on tubing.	
___	___	___	12a. Clamp tubing just as feeding is completing. Rinse tube with 30 to 60 mL warm tap water. Do not allow air to enter tubing.	
___	___	___	13a. Clamp gastric tube, and disconnect from syringe or feeding bag.	
___	___	___	14a. Have patient remain in Fowler's or elevated side-lying position for 30 to 60 minutes after feeding.	
___	___	___	15a. Wash any reusable equipment with soap and water. Change equipment every 24 hours or according to agency policy.	
___	___	___	16a. Perform hand hygiene.	
			Continuous Feeding	
___	___	___	10b. Connect feeding bag and tubing to patient's feeding tube.	
___	___	___	11b. Pour in desired amount of formula. (*Note:* Usually, hang amount of formula to infuse in 3 hours; check agency policy.) Place label on bag with patient's name, date, and time feeding was initiated.	
___	___	___	12b. Hang feeding bag on IV pole. Allow formula to flow through bag.	
___	___	___	13b. Connect tubing to infusion pump and set rate ordered by provider.	
___	___	___	14b. Patients receiving continuous feedings should have gastric residuals checked every 4 to 6 hours, according to agency policy. After checking residual and replacing stomach contents, flush the tubing with 30 to 60 mL of warm water.	
___	___	___	15b. Have patient remain in Fowler's or in slightly elevated side-lying position.	
___	___	___	16b. Wash any reusable equipment with soap and water. Change equipment every 24 hours or according to agency policy.	
___	___	___	17b. Perform hand hygiene.	
___	___	___	18b. Document appropriately.	

Procedure Checklist for Fundamentals of Nursing: Human Health and Function, 7th edition

Name ______________________ Date ______________________

Unit ______________________ Position ______________________

Instructor/Evaluator: ______________________ Position ______________________

PROCEDURE 29-1
Changing a Dry Wound Dressing

Excellent	Satisfactory	Needs Practice	**Goal:** Protect wound from trauma and external contamination; provide opportunity to assess the wound; provide an absorbent covering over the wound.	**Comments**
____	____	____	1. Perform hand hygiene and don gloves.	
____	____	____	2. Identify the patient.	
____	____	____	3. Close door or bed curtains and explain the procedure to the patient and patient's family.	
____	____	____	4. Position patient comfortably. Expose only wound area.	
____	____	____	5. Ensure that an appropriate waste receptacle is within easy reach of work area.	
____	____	____	6. Set up sterile supplies:	
____	____	____	a. Clear bedside table; wipe surface with paper towel and hand sanitizer, soap/water, or other disinfectant available.	
____	____	____	b. Open dressing package (or packages) by peeling paper down to expose dressing. Smaller dressings may be carefully dropped onto inner package of larger dressings.	
____	____	____	c. Open normal saline flush syringe packaging, or place a dermal wound cleanser spray on the table next to the open dressing packages.	
____	____	____	7. Don gloves.	
____	____	____	8. Remove dressing from wound. (*Note:* If dressing adheres to wound, apply a small amount of sterile saline on the wound to loosen the dressing.) If dressing is small, hold the dressing in the palm of one gloved hand. Remove the glove holding the dressing first, then place the first glove into the palm of the second glove. Remove the second glove.	
____	____	____	9. Dispose of gloves and old dressing in appropriate waste container. Perform hand hygiene if gloves are contaminated from wound drainage. Don clean gloves.	
____	____	____	10. Apply normal saline or spray dermal wound cleanser to the wound. Use gauze to gently cleanse wound. Cleanse around a closed incisional wound with small circular strokes to gently remove adherent wound exudates.	

Excellent	Satisfactory	Needs Practice	PROCEDURE 29-1 **Changing a Dry Wound Dressing** *(Continued)*	
___	___	___	11. Inspect the wound for bleeding, inflammation, drainage, and healing. Note any areas of dehiscence (opening or gaping of wound edges).	
___	___	___	12. Pick up sterile dressings by touching only the outer center of the dressing, and apply one at a time over the wound.	
___	___	___	13. Secure the dressings with tape. Place tape over center of dressing and evenly apply pressure to outward edges of dressings.	
___	___	___	14. Remove gloves. Perform hand hygiene.	
___	___	___	15. Document procedure.	

Procedure Checklist for Fundamentals of Nursing: Human Health and Function, 7th edition

Name ______________________ Date ______________________

Unit ______________________ Position ______________________

Instructor/Evaluator: ______________________ Position ______________________

PROCEDURE 29-2
Irrigating a Wound and Applying a Saline-Moistened Dressing

Goal: Promote moist wound healing; protect the wound from contamination and mechanical trauma.

Excellent	Satisfactory	Needs Practice		Comments
___	___	___	1. Review the provider's orders for frequency of dressing changes.	
___	___	___	2. Prepare patient and remove dressing according to steps 1 through 6 of Procedure 29-1. (*Note:* Forceps may be used to remove a soiled dressing.) If dressing adheres to underlying tissues, moisten with saline to loosen. Gently remove the dressing while assessing patient's comfort level.	
___	___	___	3. Observe dressings for amount and characteristics of drainage. Note odor and color.	
___	___	___	4. Observe wound for slough (a layer of dead cells and dried plasma, usually a yellow or yellow-brown color), granulation tissue (reddish capillary loops that bleed easily), or epithelial skin buds. Measure and record wound depth, diameter, and length.	
___	___	___	5. Place clean towel or absorbent drape pad on patient's skin adjacent to wound area.	
___	___	___	6. Don clean gloves for a chronic open wound (e.g., a pressure ulcer). Don sterile gloves for an acute full-thickness wound (e.g., dehisced surgical wound).	
___	___	___	7. Cleanse or irrigate wound as prescribed or with normal saline, moving from least to most contaminated areas. Use prefilled saline flush syringes to irrigate, or pour sterile saline from bottle into wound. Use gauze pads to cleanse wound bed and absorb excess wound exudates and irrigant solution.	
___	___	___	8. Pick up dry gauze dressings in one hand, and pour or use syringe to apply a small amount of saline onto gauze dressings. Squeeze excess fluid from gauze dressing, then unfold and fluff out the dressings.	
___	___	___	9. Check for tunneling so that all dead space can be filled. Gently fill moistened gauze into the wound cavity. If wound is deep, use forceps or cotton-tipped applicators to press gauze into all wound surfaces.	

PROCEDURE 29-2

Irrigating a Wound and Applying a Saline-Moistened Dressing *(Continued)*

Excellent	Satisfactory	Needs Practice		Comments
___	___	___	10. Apply several dry, sterile 4″ × 4″ pads over the wet gauze.	
___	___	___	11. Place ABD pad over dry 4″ × 4″ pads, if necessary.	
___	___	___	12. Dispose of gloves.	
___	___	___	13. Secure dressings with tape, Kerlix gauze (for circumferential dressings), or Montgomery ties.	
___	___	___	14. Assist patient to a comfortable position.	
___	___	___	15. Perform hand hygiene.	
___	___	___	16. Document procedure.	

Procedure Checklist for Fundamentals of Nursing: Human Health and Function, 7th edition

Name ______________________ Date ______________________

Unit ______________________ Position ______________________

Instructor/Evaluator: ______________________ Position ______________________

PROCEDURE 29-3
Maintaining a Portable Wound Suction

Goal: Facilitate healing by removing drainage from the incisional area where granulation tissue is forming.

Excellent	Satisfactory	Needs Practice	Step	Comments
____	____	____	1. Perform hand hygiene and don gloves.	
____	____	____	2. Identify the patient.	
____	____	____	3. Close door or bed curtains and explain the procedure to the patient and patient's family.	
____	____	____	4. Assist patient to a comfortable position.	
____	____	____	5. Expose wound suction tubing and container while keeping patient draped.	
____	____	____	6. Examine tubing and container for patency and suction seal. (*Note:* If the system's seal is broken, the bulb reservoir will be expanded and not compressed and suction will be lost.)	
____	____	____	7. Open the drainage plug.	
____	____	____	8. Pour drainage into a calibrated receptacle without contaminating the drainage spout. Use an antiseptic swab to clean the drainage spout.	
____	____	____	9. Reestablish suction. With drainage plug open, compress the unit and reinsert drainage plug.	
____	____	____	10. Remove and discard gloves. Perform hand hygiene.	
____	____	____	11. Return patient to a comfortable position.	
____	____	____	12. Measure drainage and record amount, color, and any other pertinent information.	
____	____	____	13. Document procedure.	

Procedure Checklist for Fundamentals of Nursing: Human Health and Function, 7th edition

Name ______________________ Date ______________

Unit ______________________ Position ______________

Instructor/Evaluator: ______________________ Position ______________

PROCEDURE 29-4

Applying a Negative-Pressure Wound Therapy Dressing

Excellent	Satisfactory	Needs Practice	**Goal:** Promote wound healing by delivering negative pressure (a vacuum) at the wound site; vacuum-assisted wound therapy helps do the following: bring wound edges together, remove wound exudates, decrease edema at wound site, develop granulation tissue.	Comments
___	___	___	1. Follow steps 1 through 5 from Procedure 29-1.	
___	___	___	2. Place towel or other protective barrier near wound and over bed linen.	
___	___	___	3. Remove dressing from wound, and discard into appropriate waste container. When removing a negative-pressure dressing, close clamp on dressing pad tubing. Disconnect dressing tubing from canister tubing. Turn off negative-pressure therapy unit. Remove dressing. If dressing adheres to wound, pour a small amount of sterile saline on the dressing and wound. It may be necessary to allow the dressing to soak for up to 15 minutes.	
___	___	___	4. Dispose of gloves; apply new pair of clean gloves (sterile gloves for acute surgical wound).	
___	___	___	5. Cleanse wound using normal saline or dermal wound cleanser and 4″ × 4″ pads.	
___	___	___	6. Measure wound—length, width, depth—and any undermined or tunneled areas using a disposable measuring guide and sterile cotton-tipped applicator.	
___	___	___	7. Dispose of gloves. Perform hand hygiene.	
___	___	___	8. Open sterile supplies (use the inside of packaging materials as sterile fields):	
___	___	___	a. Open black foam dressing kit.	
___	___	___	b. Open scissors or suture removal kit (containing scissors and forceps).	
___	___	___	c. Open skin prep wipes and place onto one of the sterile open packages.	
___	___	___	9. Don sterile gloves when applying dressing to an acute surgical wound. Don clean gloves when applying dressing to a chronically contaminated wound such as a pressure ulcer.	
___	___	___	10. Apply skin prep to 3 to 5 cm of periwound skin and allow to dry thoroughly.	

PROCEDURE 29-4

Applying a Negative-Pressure Wound Therapy Dressing *(Continued)*

Excellent	Satisfactory	Needs Practice		Comments
___	___	___	11. Cut black foam to dimensions needed to fit gently into the wound bed without overlapping onto intact periwound skin; more than one piece of black foam may be used. Do not cut black foam over the wound.	
___	___	___	12. Place black foam dressing into wound bed to gently fill wound cavity. If more than one piece of black foam is used, ensure foam to foam contact of adjacent pieces.	
___	___	___	13. Cover the foam pieces and 3 to 5 cm of periwound skin with the transparent film dressing. You may cut the drape into smaller pieces, as needed, to best fit over the wound and black foam sponge.	
___	___	___	14. Select site for connector pad; pinch the drape and cut a 2-cm round hole. Remove the backing layers from connector pad and place directly over the 2-cm hole. Apply gentle pressure to pad and peel back stabilization layer on pad.	
___	___	___	15. Insert drainage canister into negative-pressure therapy unit. Connect pad tubing to canister tubing and ensure both clamps are open.	
___	___	___	16. Turn on power to negative-pressure therapy unit; follow instructions to select prescribed therapy setting. Assess for proper seal and functioning of the negative-pressure therapy.	
___	___	___	17. Document procedure.	

Procedure Checklist for Fundamentals of Nursing: Human Health and Function, 7th edition

Name ______________________ Date ______________

Unit ______________________ Position ______________

Instructor/Evaluator: ______________________ Position ______________

PROCEDURE 29-5

Application of Heat

Excellent	Satisfactory	Needs Practice	**Goal:** Increase blood flow, resolve inflammation, improve healing of soft tissues; *or*; relieve muscular pain and stiffness; promote suppuration (discharge of purulent drainage) of indurated lesion.	Comments
___	___	___	1. Review the physician's orders to determine the type and duration of heat treatment and the treatment area.	
___	___	___	2. Perform hand hygiene.	
___	___	___	3. Identify the patient.	
___	___	___	4. Close door or bed curtains and explain the procedure to the patient.	
			Commercial Heat Pack (Variations Depending on Source of Thermotherapy)	
___	___	___	5. Remove appropriate-size pack from wrapping paper. Note the directions for squeezing and rupturing a small vessel that releases the chemical into the larger bag.	
___	___	___	6. Gently mix the bag, checking for leaks.	
___	___	___	7. Apply the pack, checking back in 3 to 5 minutes to inspect the patient's skin for erythema.	
___	___	___	8. Remove pack after 15 to 20 minutes or when it is no longer hot.	
___	___	___	9. Dispose of the heat pack. Do not reuse it.	
			Warm Moist Compress	
			Equipment	
___	___	___	1. Follow steps 1 through 4.	
___	___	___	2. Check equipment to make sure connections are secure and cords are not frayed.	
___	___	___	3. Turn pump on and set the temperature with the pump key.	
___	___	___	4. Apply warm water to washcloth or towel; wring out. Place cloth over lesion.	
___	___	___	5. Apply the pad with coiled surfaces on the warm moist cloth.	
___	___	___	6. Secure with tape, if needed.	
___	___	___	7. Check the patient's skin and area of treatment every 10 minutes for the first 20 minutes to be sure the temperature is well tolerated. Discontinue compress after 30 minutes.	
___	___	___	8. Check water level on aquathermia unit to make sure it is at the appropriate level.	
___	___	___	9. Document procedure.	

Procedure Checklist for Fundamentals of Nursing: Human Health and Function, 7th edition

Name ______________________ Date ______________________

Unit ______________________ Position ______________________

Instructor/Evaluator: ______________________ Position ______________________

PROCEDURE 29-6

Application of Cold

Excellent	Satisfactory	Needs Practice	**Goal:** Relieve swelling and inflammation and decrease bleeding; promote patient comfort in first 24 hours after an acute injury.	Comments
____	____	____	1. Review the provider's order to determine the duration of cold treatment and the treatment area.	
____	____	____	2. Perform hand hygiene and don gloves.	
____	____	____	3. Identify the patient.	
____	____	____	4. Close door or bed curtains and explain the procedure to the patient and patient's family.	
____	____	____	5. Fill ice bag with crushed/cubed ice to fill line; clamp bag closed. If not using commercially prepared bag, cover plastic bag with cloth.	
____	____	____	6. Apply the pack, and use ties to keep cold application to desired location. Check back in 5 minutes to inspect the patient's skin for coldness or numbness.	
____	____	____	7. Remove bag after 15 to 20 minutes. Reapply fresh ice bag in 1 to 2 hours as needed.	
____	____	____	8. Document procedure.	

Procedure Checklist for Fundamentals of Nursing: Human Health and Function, 7th edition

Name ______________________ Date ______________

Unit ______________________ Position ______________

Instructor/Evaluator: ______________________ Position ______________

PROCEDURE 30-1
Obtaining a Wound Culture

Goal: Identify organisms colonized within a wound so that antibiotics sensitive to the microorganisms can be prescribed, as needed.

Excellent	Satisfactory	Needs Practice		Comments
___	___	___	1. Identify the patient using two separate identifiers.	
___	___	___	2. Close door or bed curtains and explain the procedure to the patient, if possible.	
___	___	___	3. Verify order for culture noting site and type of culture. Label the specimen container and make sure the information includes the patient's name, medical record number, date and time specimen is obtained, and site of the culture.	
___	___	___	4. Perform hand hygiene and don gloves.	
___	___	___	5. Remove soiled dressing. Observe drainage for amount, odor, and color.	
___	___	___	6. Clear and remove exudate from around wound and cleanse with normal saline.	
			Obtaining Aerobic Culture	
___	___	___	1. Perform steps 1 through 6 above.	
___	___	___	2. Using sterile swab from culture tube, insert swab deep into area of active drainage. Rotate swab to absorb as much drainage as possible.	
___	___	___	3. Insert swab into culture tube, taking care not to touch the top or outside of the tube.	
___	___	___	4. Crush ampule of medium and close container securely.	
___	___	___	5. Continue with step 4 below.	
			Obtaining Anaerobic Culture	
___	___	___	1. Perform steps 1 through 6 at beginning of procedure.	
___	___	___	2. Using sterile swab from special anaerobic culture tube, insert swab deeply into draining body cavity.	
___	___	___	3. a. Rotate swab gently and remove. Quickly place swab into inner tube of collection container.	
___	___	___	b. *Alternative method:* Insert tip of syringe with needle removed into wound and aspirate 1 to 5 mL of exudate. Attach 21-gauge needle to syringe, expel all air, and inject exudate into inner tube of the culture container.	

Excellent	Satisfactory	Needs Practice	PROCEDURE 30-1 **Obtaining a Wound Culture** *(Continued)*	Comments
___	___	___	4. Send specimens in the prelabeled containers with appropriate requisition immediately to the laboratory. Some agencies require that specimens be transported in clean plastic bags to further prevent transfer of microorganisms.	
___	___	___	5. Clean and apply sterile dressings to the wound, as ordered.	
___	___	___	6. Remove and discard gloves. Perform hand hygiene.	
___	___	___	7. Document all relevant information on the patient's chart. Include the location the specimen was taken from and the date and time. Record the wound's appearance and the color, odor, amount, and consistency of drainage. Record how the patient tolerated the procedure and any discomfort that he or she experienced.	

Procedure Checklist for Fundamentals of Nursing: Human Health and Function, 7th edition

Name ______________________ Date ______________________

Unit ______________________ Position ______________________

Instructor/Evaluator: ______________________ Position ______________________

PROCEDURE 31-1

Assessing Urine Volume Using a Bladder Ultrasonic Scanner

Excellent	Satisfactory	Needs Practice	**Goal:** To noninvasively calculate the volume of urine in the bladder; to determine the need for catheterization to relieve urinary retention.	Comments
___	___	___	1. Perform hand hygiene and don gloves.	
___	___	___	2. Identify the patient with two separate identifiers (name, medical record number, date of birth).	
___	___	___	3. Close door or bed curtains and explain procedure to the patient.	
___	___	___	4. Raise the bed to a comfortable working height. Assist the patient to lie as flat as can be tolerated comfortably. Expose only the patient's lower abdomen and suprapubic area.	
___	___	___	5. Clean scan head probe (sound wave transducer) with isopropyl alcohol.	
___	___	___	6. Turn the bladder scanner on and press "scan."	
___	___	___	7. Press "male" or "female" mode on scan device. If a female patient has had a hysterectomy (removal of uterus), press "male."	
___	___	___	8. Gently palpate the patient's symphysis pubis and then apply ultrasound gel midline on the abdomen (about 1 to 1.5 inches above the symphysis pubis), or apply ultrasound gel directly to the scan head.	
___	___	___	9. Find the symphysis pubis (midline below the umbilicus) and place the scan head approximately 3 cm superior to the symphysis pubis, pointing toward the expected bladder location. Locate the icon on the scan head and point the icon toward the patient's head.	
___	___	___	10. Press the scan head button and hold the scan head steady until a beep is heard, then release.	
___	___	___	11. The bladder scan will display the bladder volume measurement and an aiming display. Adjust scan head aim to obtain intersection of the crosshair and the bladder. Reposition the scan head and repeat the measurement as needed to obtain a centered image.	

PROCEDURE 31-1

Assessing Urine Volume Using a Bladder Ultrasonic Scanner *(Continued)*

Excellent	Satisfactory	Needs Practice		Comments
___	___	___	12. When finished, press "done" and print for a hard copy of results.	
___	___	___	13. Wipe gel from patient's skin and reposition patient if needed.	
___	___	___	14. Dispose of contaminated supplies. Clean scan head with isopropyl alcohol. Perform hand hygiene.	
___	___	___	15. Document urine volumes obtained via BUS.	

Procedure Checklist for Fundamentals of Nursing: Human Health and Function, 7th edition

Name ______________________ Date ______________________

Unit ______________________ Position ______________________

Instructor/Evaluator: ______________________ Position ______________________

PROCEDURE 31-2

Collecting Urine Specimens

Goal: Obtain a noncontaminated urine specimen for routine analysis or culture and sensitivity.

				Comments
___	___	___	1. Confirm the physician's order.	
___	___	___	2. Perform hand hygiene and don gloves.	
___	___	___	3. Identify the patient with two separate identifiers (name, medical record number, date of birth).	
___	___	___	4. Close door or bed curtains and explain procedure to the patient.	
			Collecting Sterile Specimen From an Indwelling Catheter	
___	___	___	5. Position patient so that catheter is accessible.	
___	___	___	6. Drain urine from tubing into collection bag. Allow fresh urine to collect in tubing by clamping or bending tubing (2 mL of urine is sufficient for a culture and sensitivity specimen, 30 mL for urinalysis).	
___	___	___	7. Cleanse the aspiration port of the drainage tubing with alcohol or antimicrobial swab.	
___	___	___	8. Insert syringe into aspiration port. Draw urine sample into syringe by gentle aspiration. Remove syringe from port and unclamp the drainage tubing.	
___	___	___	9. Transfer urine from syringe into a sterile specimen container.	
___	___	___	10. Identify the patient with at least two identifiers (name, medical record number, birth date) and match this information to the label on the container. Note date and time on laboratory requisition form. Place in plastic biohazard bag for delivery to the laboratory.	
___	___	___	11. Send specimen to laboratory within 15 minutes or place in specimen refrigerator. If specimen is for microbiology testing, it must be sent immediately and not refrigerated.	
___	___	___	12. Dispose of all contaminated supplies. Perform hand hygiene.	
___	___	___	13. Document procedure and observations.	

Excellent	Satisfactory	Needs Practice	PROCEDURE 31-2 **Collecting Urine Specimens** *(Continued)*	Comments
			Self-Collecting Midstream Urine Specimen for a Woman	
___	___	___	1. Follow steps 1 through 4.	
___	___	___	2. Give the patient the following instructions on how to cleanse urinary meatus and obtain a urine specimen:	
___	___	___	a. Perform hand hygiene.	
___	___	___	b. Separate labia minora and cleanse perineum with commercially prepared aseptic swabs, starting in front of the urethral meatus and moving swab toward the rectum.	
___	___	___	c. Repeat this cleansing process three times with different cotton balls or swabs.	
___	___	___	d. Begin to urinate while continuing to hold labia apart. Allow first urine to flow into toilet.	
___	___	___	e. Hold specimen container under the urine stream.	
___	___	___	f. Remove specimen container, release hand from labia, seal container tightly, and finish voiding; perform hand hygiene.	
___	___	___	3. Put on disposable gloves to receive specimen container from the patient. Dry outside of container with a paper towel.	
___	___	___	4. Date and time laboratory specimen. Verify the patient by two identifiers and make sure they match the label. Label the container and place specimen container in biohazard bag.	
___	___	___	5. Send specimen to laboratory within 15 minutes or place in specimen refrigerator. If specimen is for microbiology testing, it must be sent immediately and not refrigerated.	
___	___	___	6. Dispose of all contaminated supplies. Wash hands.	
			Self-Collecting Midstream Urine Specimen for a Man	
___	___	___	1. Follow steps 1 through 4.	
___	___	___	2. Give the patient the following instructions on how to cleanse urinary meatus and obtain urine specimen:	
___	___	___	a. Perform hand hygiene.	
___	___	___	b. Starting at the top in a circular motion, cleanse end of penis with cotton balls and soap or commercially prepared antiseptic swabs. If the man is not circumcised, he should retract his foreskin to expose the urinary meatus before cleansing and throughout specimen collection.	
___	___	___	c. Repeat cleansing three times with three separate cotton balls or antiseptic swabs.	
___	___	___	d. Begin to urinate, allowing first urine to flow into toilet.	
___	___	___	e. Pass specimen container into urine stream.	
___	___	___	f. Remove container, seal tightly, and finish voiding.	

PROCEDURE 31-2

Collecting Urine Specimens *(Continued)*

Excellent	Satisfactory	Needs Practice		Comments
___	___	___	3. Follow steps 3 through 6 above under the Self-Collecting Midstream Urine Specimen for a Woman section.	
			Collecting a Specimen From a Child Without Urinary Control	
___	___	___	1. Follow steps 1 through 4.	
___	___	___	2. If parents are present, explain procedure to them.	
___	___	___	3. Position child gently on his or her back. Put on disposable gloves. Remove diaper.	
___	___	___	4. *For a girl:* Clean perineal–genital area gently with soap and water, followed by antiseptic. Separate labia and cleanse from front of urethral meatus toward the rectum. Rinse with water and dry with cotton balls.	
___	___	___	5. *For a boy:* Clean perineal–genital area gently with soap and water, followed by antiseptic. Cleanse the penis and scrotum. If the boy is not circumcised, retract the foreskin and cleanse. Rinse with water and dry with gauze or cotton balls.	
___	___	___	6. Remove paper backing from adhesive of collection bag.	
___	___	___	7. Spread the child's legs widely apart.	
___	___	___	8. Apply collection bag over child's perineum, covering penis and scrotum of a boy, urinary meatus and vagina of a girl. Press adhesive to secure, starting at the perineum and working outward.	
___	___	___	9. Place a diaper on the child loosely.	
___	___	___	10. Remove gloves and perform hand hygiene.	
___	___	___	11. Check the collector for urine every 15 minutes. Parents can check child for urine specimen.	
___	___	___	12. When urine specimen is obtained, glove again, gently remove collection bag from the skin, and empty urine into specimen container.	
___	___	___	13. Tighten lid, cleanse outside of container if contaminated with urine, and place in plastic biohazard bag for transfer to the laboratory.	
___	___	___	14. Label the container, making sure that patient information is correct. Record date and time on laboratory requisition form.	
___	___	___	15. Send specimen to laboratory within 15 minutes or place in specimen refrigerator. If specimen is for microbiology testing, it must be sent immediately and not refrigerated.	
___	___	___	16. Dispose of all contaminated supplies. Perform hand hygiene.	
___	___	___	17. Document that specimen was collected and sent.	

Procedure Checklist for Fundamentals of Nursing: Human Health and Function, 7th edition

Name ______________________ Date ______________________

Unit ______________________ Position ______________________

Instructor/Evaluator: ______________________ Position ______________________

PROCEDURE 31-3
Applying an External Catheter

Goal: Provide a means of collecting urine and controlling incontinence with less risk of infection that an indwelling urinary catheter imposes.

Excellent	Satisfactory	Needs Practice		Comments
____	____	____	1. Perform hand hygiene.	
____	____	____	2. Identify the patient.	
____	____	____	3. Close door or bed curtains and explain procedure to the patient.	
____	____	____	4. Raise the bed to a comfortable working height. Assist patient to supine position with thighs slightly apart. Drape patient so that only the area around the genitalia is exposed.	
____	____	____	5. Put on disposable gloves. Wash patient's genitals with plain soap and water. Clean the tip of the penis first using a circular motion from the meatus outward. Wash the shaft of the penis using downward strokes toward the pubic area. Towel dry. For an uncircumcised male, retract the foreskin and clean the glans of the penis. Be sure to replace the foreskin after cleansing.	
____	____	____	6. Trim excess pubic hair from base of penis using blunt-end scissors, if necessary.	
____	____	____	7. If not using a self-adhesive sheath, apply thin film of skin protector supplied in kit on penis shaft. Allow to dry for 30 seconds.	
____	____	____	8. Grasp penis firmly with nondominant hand. Apply sheath by guiding opening over the glans of the penis and then unrolling the sheath the length of the penis using dominant hand. Leave only a small gap between the tip of the penis and the drainage port of the sheath. Gently press sheath to shaft of penis to secure adhesive inside the catheter to the skin.	
____	____	____	9. Attach drainage port of the sheath to collection system tubing. Avoid kinks or loops in the tubing. Secure drainage tubing to patient's abdomen or inner thigh with securement device.	
____	____	____	10. Discard used supplies and perform hand hygiene.	
____	____	____	11. Assist patient to a comfortable position and cover him with bed linens. Place the bed in the lowest position.	

PROCEDURE 31-3

Applying an External Catheter *(Continued)*

Excellent	Satisfactory	Needs Practice		Comments
___	___	___	12. Secure collection system bag below the level of the bladder. Check that the tubing is not kinked and that movement of bed rails does not interfere with the drainage system.	
___	___	___	13. Observe penis 15 to 30 minutes after application of condom for swelling or changes in skin color. Routinely remove external catheter, examine the underlying skin, and reapply at least every 24 hours or if patient complains of any discomfort.	
___	___	___	14. Document application and removal of external catheter and the condition of the skin.	

Procedure Checklist for Fundamentals of Nursing: Human Health and Function, 7th edition

Name ______________________________ Date ______________________

Unit ______________________________ Position ______________________

Instructor/Evaluator: ______________________________ Position ______________________

PROCEDURE 31-4

Inserting a Straight or Indwelling Urinary Catheter

Excellent	Satisfactory	Needs Practice	Goal: **Indwelling Catheterization:** monitor urinary function; prevent or relieve bladder distention; provide continuous bladder drainage; provide a means for irrigating the bladder with fluids or medication; **Straight or Intermittent Catheterization:** obtain sterile urine specimens; routine emptying of the bladder in patients with neurogenic bladder; measure residual urine.	Comments
			Initial Steps for Inserting Straight or Indwelling Catheters	
____	____	____	1. Confirm the physician's order.	
____	____	____	2. Perform hand hygiene and don gloves.	
____	____	____	3. Identify the patient with two separate identifiers (name, medical record number, date of birth).	
____	____	____	4. Determine if patient has any allergies (especially to iodine and latex).	
____	____	____	5. Close door or bed curtains and explain procedure to the patient.	
____	____	____	6. Set up good light source. Place trash receptacle within easy reach.	
____	____	____	7. Raise the bed to a comfortable working height. Stand on the patient's right side if you are right-handed, on the patient's left side if you are left-handed.	
____	____	____	8. Provide the patient with opportunity to perform personal perineal/penile hygiene. If the patient is unable or unwilling to perform personal hygiene, assist or perform hygiene as necessary. Slide waterproof pad under patient. For the female patient, wipe from front to back. For the male patient, clean the tip of the penis first, using circular motions from the meatus outward, and then cleanse the shaft of the penis using downward strokes toward the pubic area. Remove gloves and perform hand hygiene.	
			Inserting an Indwelling Catheter in a Female Patient	
____	____	____	9. Position patient in dorsal recumbent position (supine with knees flexed). Externally rotate thighs. Side-lying is an alternative position.	

Excellent	Satisfactory	Needs Practice	PROCEDURE 31-4 **Inserting a Straight or Indwelling Urinary Catheter** *(Continued)*	Comments
___	___	___	10. Open the catheterization tray on clean bedside table while maintaining asepsis. See Procedure 18-3 for preparing and maintaining a sterile field. If necessary, put on clean gloves. Pick up drape from the top of the catheterization kit, touching only the corners of the drape. Slide sterile drape under patient's buttocks; ask patient to lift hips if possible so drape can be slid under easily. Do not touch center of drape.	
___	___	___	11. If used, remove clean gloves. Don sterile gloves. Place fenestrated sterile drape over the perineal area. Place sterile catheterization tray on sterile drape between patient's thighs.	
___	___	___	12. Open sterile lubricant and lubricate the catheter tip. With a physician's order, 2% lidocaine gel can also be used for lubrication. Open cleansing solution and pour over half of the sterile balls or open antimicrobial cleansing swabs. Open the sterile specimen container. Do not test inflate the balloon.	
___	___	___	13. Place nondominant hand on labia minora and gently spread to expose urinary meatus. (This hand is now considered contaminated.) Visualize exact location of meatus. During cleansing and catheter insertion, do not allow labia to close over meatus until after the catheter is inserted.	
___	___	___	14. Using sterile hand, pick up saturated cotton ball with sterile forceps or antimicrobial swabs.	
___	___	___	15. Cleanse the urinary meatus with a downward stroke. Discard the cotton ball or antimicrobial swab. Repeat this step three or four times.	
___	___	___	16. Use dry cotton balls to absorb excess antiseptic solution.	
___	___	___	17. With sterile hand, pick up the catheter approximately 3 inches from the tip and place distal catheter end into sterile basin. If the catheter is attached to sterile tubing and drainage container (closed drainage system), position catheter and setup within easy reach on the sterile field. Make sure clamp on drainage bag is closed.	
___	___	___	18. Gently insert catheter into urethra (approximately 2 inches) until urine begins to drain. If no urine appears, have patient cough or reposition catheter by rotating. Have patient take slow, deep breaths during catheter insertion.	
___	___	___	19. Insert the catheter an additional 1 inch (2.5 cm).	
___	___	___	20. Inflate the retention balloon with the prefilled syringe. Check to ensure placement by gently pulling on catheter.	

PROCEDURE 31-4

Inserting a Straight or Indwelling Urinary Catheter *(Continued)*

Excellent	Satisfactory	Needs Practice		Comments
___	___	___	21. Connect distal end of catheter to drainage bag. In some kits, the catheter is already connected to the drainage unit. Some nurses prefer to connect equipment before catheter insertion.	
___	___	___	22. Secure catheter tubing to the patient's inner thigh with Velcro leg strap or other securement device, with enough give so that it will not pull when the legs move.	
___	___	___	23. Attach drainage bag to bed frame, ensuring that tubing does not fall into dependent loops and that side rails do not interfere with drainage system.	
___	___	___	24. Remove gloves and perform hand hygiene.	
___	___	___	25. Record the time of completion of the procedure, size of catheter inserted, amount and color of urine, and any adverse patient responses.	
			Inserting a Straight Catheter in a Female Patient	
___	___	___	1. Follow steps 1 through 18.	
___	___	___	2. With sterile hand, place the drainage end of the catheter in a receptacle. If a specimen is required, place the end into the specimen container in the receptacle.	
___	___	___	3. Gently insert catheter into urethra (approximately 2 inches) until urine begins to drain. If no urine appears, have patient cough or reposition catheter by rotating. Have patient take slow, deep breaths during catheter insertion.	
___	___	___	4. Hold the catheter securely at the urinary meatus while the bladder empties. If ordered, obtain urine specimen in sterile container, pinching catheter once specimen is obtained. Add volume of specimen to the residual volume obtained.	
___	___	___	5. Allow the bladder to empty completely. Withdraw the catheter slowly and smoothly. Wash and dry genital area as necessary.	
___	___	___	6. Remove gloves and assist patient to a comfortable position. Cover the patient with a gown and bed linens.	
___	___	___	7. Put on clean gloves. Cover and label urine specimen if applicable and place in plastic bag with lab requisition form. Check patient identity with two separate identifiers. Send urine specimen to the laboratory immediately.	
___	___	___	8. Remove gloves and perform hand hygiene.	

PROCEDURE 31-4

Inserting a Straight or Indwelling Urinary Catheter *(Continued)*

Excellent	Satisfactory	Needs Practice		Comments
			Inserting an Indwelling Catheter in a Male Patient	
___	___	___	9. Position patient in supine position with only genitalia exposed.	
___	___	___	10. Drape legs to midthigh with bath blanket or sheet.	
___	___	___	11. Open the sterile catheterization tray on a clean bedside table, maintaining asepsis.	
___	___	___	12. Put on sterile gloves. Place the fenestrated drape over the patient's genitalia. Place sterile catheterization tray between patient's legs on the sterile drape.	
___	___	___	13. Open cleansing solution and pour over half of the sterile cotton balls, or open antimicrobial swabs. Open the sterile specimen container. Do not test inflate the balloon.	
___	___	___	14. Using sterile hand, place the distal catheter end into sterile basin. If catheter is preattached to sterile tubing and drainage container (closed drainage system), position catheter and setup within easy reach on sterile field. Ensure that clamp on drainage bag is closed. Remove cap from syringe prefilled with lubricant and squirt onto sterile field.	
___	___	___	15. With your nondominant hand, hold the penis at a 90-degree angle to the body. If the patient is not circumcised, pull back the foreskin with this hand to visualize the urethral meatus. (This hand is now considered unsterile.)	
___	___	___	16. Using the sterile hand, pick up the cleansing solution—either antimicrobial swabs or the soaked cotton ball (using sterile forceps).	
___	___	___	17. Cleanse the urinary meatus with one downward stroke or use a circular motion from meatus to base of penis. Discard the cotton ball or antimicrobial swabs. Repeat this step at least three or four times.	
___	___	___	18. Use forceps to pick up one dry cotton ball to dry the meatus.	
___	___	___	19. Hold penis with slight upward tension and perpendicular to the patient's body. Lubricate catheter well with lubricant or lidocaine. For a patient needing extra lubrication, the lubricant or lidocaine can be injected directly into the penis.	
___	___	___	20. Gently insert catheter into urethra (approximately 8 inches) until urine begins to drain.	
___	___	___	21. Insert catheter an additional 1 inch (2.5 cm).	
___	___	___	22. Inflate the balloon with the prefilled syringe.	
___	___	___	23. Check for placement by gently pulling on catheter.	

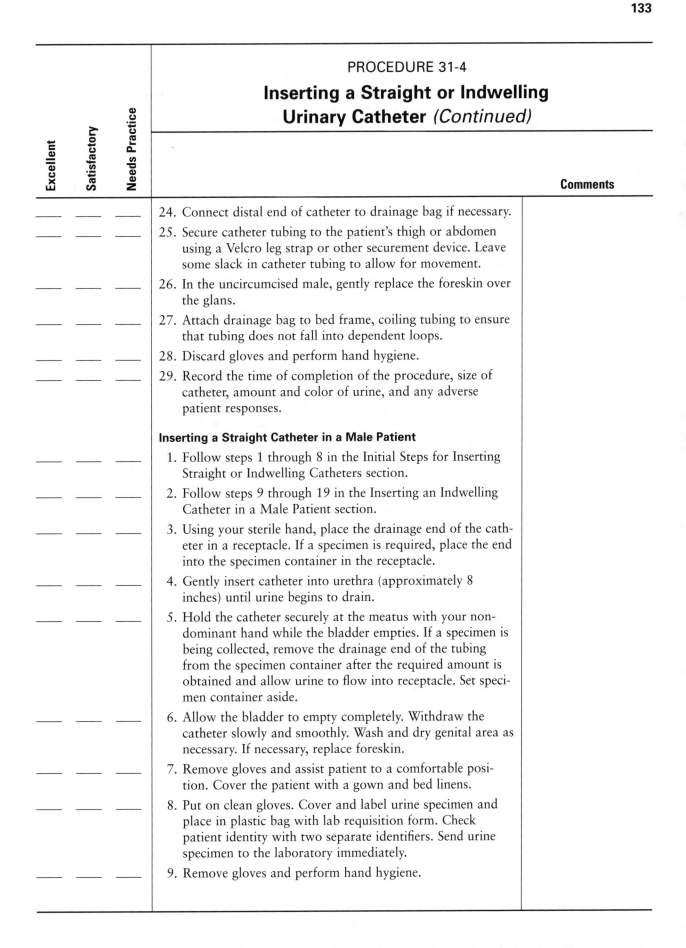

PROCEDURE 31-4

Inserting a Straight or Indwelling Urinary Catheter *(Continued)*

Excellent	Satisfactory	Needs Practice		Comments
___	___	___	24. Connect distal end of catheter to drainage bag if necessary.	
___	___	___	25. Secure catheter tubing to the patient's thigh or abdomen using a Velcro leg strap or other securement device. Leave some slack in catheter tubing to allow for movement.	
___	___	___	26. In the uncircumcised male, gently replace the foreskin over the glans.	
___	___	___	27. Attach drainage bag to bed frame, coiling tubing to ensure that tubing does not fall into dependent loops.	
___	___	___	28. Discard gloves and perform hand hygiene.	
___	___	___	29. Record the time of completion of the procedure, size of catheter, amount and color of urine, and any adverse patient responses.	
			Inserting a Straight Catheter in a Male Patient	
___	___	___	1. Follow steps 1 through 8 in the Initial Steps for Inserting Straight or Indwelling Catheters section.	
___	___	___	2. Follow steps 9 through 19 in the Inserting an Indwelling Catheter in a Male Patient section.	
___	___	___	3. Using your sterile hand, place the drainage end of the catheter in a receptacle. If a specimen is required, place the end into the specimen container in the receptacle.	
___	___	___	4. Gently insert catheter into urethra (approximately 8 inches) until urine begins to drain.	
___	___	___	5. Hold the catheter securely at the meatus with your non-dominant hand while the bladder empties. If a specimen is being collected, remove the drainage end of the tubing from the specimen container after the required amount is obtained and allow urine to flow into receptacle. Set specimen container aside.	
___	___	___	6. Allow the bladder to empty completely. Withdraw the catheter slowly and smoothly. Wash and dry genital area as necessary. If necessary, replace foreskin.	
___	___	___	7. Remove gloves and assist patient to a comfortable position. Cover the patient with a gown and bed linens.	
___	___	___	8. Put on clean gloves. Cover and label urine specimen and place in plastic bag with lab requisition form. Check patient identity with two separate identifiers. Send urine specimen to the laboratory immediately.	
___	___	___	9. Remove gloves and perform hand hygiene.	

PROCEDURE 31-4

Inserting a Straight or Indwelling Urinary Catheter *(Continued)*

Excellent	Satisfactory	Needs Practice		Comments
			Removing an Indwelling Catheter	
___	___	___	1. Follow steps 1 through 4.	
___	___	___	2. Position patient as for catheter insertion. Drape patient so that only the area around the catheter is exposed. Place a waterproof pad under the female patient's legs or over the male patient's thighs.	
___	___	___	3. Clamp the catheter (optional).	
___	___	___	4. Remove the securement device used to secure the catheter tubing to the patient's thigh or abdomen.	
___	___	___	5. Insert hub of syringe into balloon inflation tube of catheter and allow syringe to fill with liquid from balloon. Do not pull on syringe to withdraw liquid. Size of balloon is indicated on catheter; most commonly, sizes smaller than 10 mL are used. Larger balloons (30 mL) may be used after prostatic or urologic surgery.	
___	___	___	6. Ask patient to breathe in and out deeply. Pinch catheter and remove slowly and gently as patient exhales.	
___	___	___	7. Place catheter on waterproof pad and wrap in pad.	
___	___	___	8. Assist patient to cleanse and dry genitals. Remove gloves and assist patient to a comfortable position. Place gown over patient and cover the patient with bed linens.	
___	___	___	9. Put on clean gloves. Remove and dispose of used equipment according to agency policy. Measure and document urine in drainage bag and time of catheter removal. Estimate when patient should void (within 8 hours).	
___	___	___	10. Remove gloves and perform hand hygiene.	
___	___	___	11. Document the time of catheter removal, time patient should void, and any adverse signs or symptoms.	

Procedure Checklist for Fundamentals of Nursing: Human Health and Function, 7th edition

Name ______________________ Date ______________

Unit ______________________ Position ______________

Instructor/Evaluator: ______________________ Position ______________

PROCEDURE 32-1

Assessing Stool for Occult Blood

Excellent	Satisfactory	Needs Practice	**Goal:** Screen patients who have or who are at risk for gastrointestinal bleeding; screen for early-stage colon cancer.	**Comments**
___	___	___	1. Perform hand hygiene.	
___	___	___	2. Identify the patient.	
___	___	___	3. Close door or bed curtains and explain procedure to the patient.	
___	___	___	4. Ask the patient to void before collecting the stool specimen.	
___	___	___	5. Assist patient onto bedpan or commode or to bathroom. Provide privacy; leave call bell handy.	
___	___	___	6. Once the patient has passed stool and is clean and comfortable, don disposable gloves and obtain small amount of stool with a tongue blade or wooden applicator.	
			Hemoccult Slide Test	
___	___	___	7. Open flap of slide and apply a very thin smear of stool taken from the center of the specimen onto first window.	
___	___	___	8. Using second applicator, obtain a second sample from a different area of the stool. Smear thinly on second window of slide.	
___	___	___	9. Wait 3 minutes.	
___	___	___	10. Close slide cover and turn over. Then open flap on reverse side and apply two drops of the developing solution onto each window and one drop onto control window. Wait 30 to 60 seconds. Read test results.	
___	___	___	11. Remove gloves, wash hands, and document findings.	

Procedure Checklist for Fundamentals of Nursing: Human Health and Function, 7th edition

Name ______________________ Date ______________________

Unit ______________________ Position ______________________

Instructor/Evaluator: ______________________ Position ______________________

PROCEDURE 32-2
Administering an Enema

Excellent	Satisfactory	Needs Practice	**Goal:** Relieves gas, constipation, or fecal impaction; cleanses the bowel in preparation for diagnostic tests or surgical procedures; evacuates feces in patients with hemiplegia, quadriplegia, or paraplegia; delivers medication.	**Comments**
			Large-Volume Enema	
___	___	___	1. Assemble the needed equipment in one place.	
___	___	___	2. Prepare solution. Check temperature of solution by pouring some over your inner wrist. Fill enema bag with 750 to 1,000 mL lukewarm solution (105° to 110°F; for child, 500 mL or less, 100°F).	
___	___	___	3. Open clamp on tubing and allow solution to flow through tubing to remove the air. Reclamp tubing.	
___	___	___	4. Provide privacy by closing curtains or room door.	
___	___	___	5. Identify patient. Position patient on left side (Sims' position) with right knee flexed.	
___	___	___	6. Cover patient with bath blanket, exposing only the buttocks.	
___	___	___	7. Put on disposable gloves. Place waterproof pad under patient's buttocks.	
___	___	___	8. Lubricate 2 to 3 inches of the tip of the rectal tube with water-soluble lubricant.	
___	___	___	9. Separate the buttocks to visualize the anus. Observe for external hemorrhoids. Ask patient to take a slow, deep breath. Gently insert the tube, directing the tip toward the umbilicus (adult: 3 to 4 inches).	
___	___	___	10. Continue holding the tube in the rectum. With other hand, open the clamp and allow solution to slowly enter the patient. Raise container 18 inches above the anus, allowing solution to flow slowly over 5 to 10 minutes; if patient complains of cramping or pain, have patient breathe deeply and lower bag until the sensation stops.	
___	___	___	11. Reclamp tubing when desired amount of solution has infused.	
___	___	___	12. Remove tube gently and have patient squeeze buttocks together firmly for several minutes.	
___	___	___	13. Have patient retain solution as long as possible.	

PROCEDURE 32-2
Administering an Enema *(Continued)*

Excellent	Satisfactory	Needs Practice		Comments
___	___	___	14. Assist patient to bathroom, commode, or bedpan. Place call bell within reach. Provide privacy until all of the solution has been expelled.	
___	___	___	15. Visually inspect character of the feces and solution.	
___	___	___	16. Assist patient into comfortable position. Assist with cleansing as needed. Provide materials for patient to wash hands. Open windows or provide air freshener if needed. Clean and dispose of equipment as necessary. Remove gloves and wash hands.	
			Small-Volume Enema	
___	___	___	1. Assemble the needed equipment in one place.	
___	___	___	2. Provide privacy by closing curtains or room door.	
___	___	___	3. Identify patient. Position patient on left side (Sims' position) with right knee flexed.	
___	___	___	4. Put on disposable gloves. Place waterproof towel under patient's buttocks.	
___	___	___	5. Cover patient with bath blanket, exposing only the buttocks.	
___	___	___	6. Remove protective cap from prelubricated catheter tip. You may add more lubricant if necessary.	
___	___	___	7. Separate the buttocks to visualize the anus. Observe for hemorrhoids and gently insert rectal tip into rectum, directing the tip toward the umbilicus.	
___	___	___	8. Squeeze bottle to empty contents into the rectum and colon (approximately 240 mL of solution).	
___	___	___	9. Maintain pressure on the enema container until you withdraw it from the rectum.	
___	___	___	10. Continue with steps 13 through 16 above for a large-volume enema.	
___	___	___	11. Document administration and the results from the enema.	

Procedure Checklist for Fundamentals of Nursing: Human Health and Function, 7th edition

Name ______________________ Date ______________________

Unit ______________________ Position ______________________

Instructor/Evaluator: ______________________ Position ______________________

PROCEDURE 32-3

Applying a Fecal Ostomy Pouch

Excellent	Satisfactory	Needs Practice	**Goal:** Contains drainage and odors for the comfort of the patient and allows accurate assessment of output; protects the peristomal skin from excoriation; allows accurate assessment of output, especially in the postoperative period; provides visualization of the stoma and sutures during the postoperative period.	Comments
___	___	___	1. Perform hand hygiene and don gloves. The patient may perform the procedure without gloves.	
___	___	___	2. Identify the patient.	
___	___	___	3. Close door or bed curtains and explain procedure to the patient.	
___	___	___	4. Place a waterproof pad by stoma site.	
___	___	___	5. Gently remove old appliance (and skin barrier if applicable) by pushing skin away from appliance (do not pull appliance from skin); start at the top of the appliance. If disposable, discard. If reusable, set aside for washing.	
___	___	___	6. Use toilet tissue to remove excess stool. Wash skin thoroughly around stoma with skin cleanser or soap and water.	
___	___	___	7. Rinse skin thoroughly and blot dry.	
___	___	___	8. Observe condition of peristomal skin, the stoma, and the sutures. Teach the patient to make these observations daily.	
___	___	___	9. Cover stoma with gauze while you prepare new appliance. Prepare appliance and/or skin barrier: Measure stoma using a measurement guide, and trace stoma measurement on the adhesive paper backing of appliance or barrier. Cut the opening ⅛ inch larger than tracing.	
___	___	___	10. If stoma is located in an abdominal crease or the skin is irregular, use a paste barrier to fill the irregularity.	
___	___	___	11. Apply protectant as needed/desired. Allow protectant to dry completely.	
___	___	___	12. Apply protective skin barrier:	
___	___	___	a. Peel paper backing off wafer, and center stoma in hole.	
___	___	___	b. Place on abdomen, pressing lightly over all areas of the barrier to promote adhesion with skin surfaces.	

PROCEDURE 32-3

Applying a Fecal Ostomy Pouch *(Continued)*

Excellent	Satisfactory	Needs Practice		Comments
____	____	____	13. Attach drainable pouch to skin barrier. Some equipment attaches by means of a plastic flange that snaps in place; other models adhere through self-adherent tape that is exposed after protective paper backing is removed. Tug gently or inspect for secure fit.	
____	____	____	14. Fold over bottom edge of pouch and clamp.	
____	____	____	15. Dispose of old appliance. Clean and store any reusable supplies. Wash hands. Document observations.	

Procedure Checklist for Fundamentals of Nursing: Human Health and Function, 7th edition

Name ______________________ Date ______________________

Unit ______________________ Position ______________________

Instructor/Evaluator: ______________________ Position ______________________

PROCEDURE 32-4

Inserting a Nasogastric Tube

Goal: Decompresses the stomach to relieve pressure and prevent vomiting; provides a means for irrigating the stomach (lavage); provides access to gastric specimens for laboratory analysis; provides a route for delivering liquid enteral feedings (gavage) in patients who can't swallow or ingest adequate calorie intake (see Chapter 28).

Excellent	Satisfactory	Needs Practice	Step	Comments
___	___	___	1. Perform hand hygiene.	
___	___	___	2. Identify the patient.	
___	___	___	3. Close door or bed curtains and explain procedure to the patient. Insertion is not painful, but it is uncomfortable because the gag reflex is usually stimulated.	
___	___	___	4. Raise bed to high Fowler's position, cover chest with towel or drape, and place emesis basin nearby.	
___	___	___	5. Determine length of tubing to be inserted by measuring nasogastric tube from tip of nose to tip of earlobe, then to tip of xiphoid process. Mark tubing with adhesive tape or note striped markings already on the tube.	
___	___	___	6. Put on gloves. Lubricate tip of tube with water-soluble lubricant.	
___	___	___	7. Gently insert tube into nostril. Advance toward posterior pharynx.	
___	___	___	8. Have patient tilt head forward and encourage patient to drink water slowly. Advance tube without using force as patient swallows. Advance tube until desired insertion length is reached.	
___	___	___	9. Temporarily tape the tube to the patient's nose, then assess placement of the tube:	
___	___	___	a. Aspirate gastric content with 20- to 50-mL syringe; note color and test pH. If the pH is 5 or less, it can be assumed that the tube is in the stomach.	
___	___	___	b. If feeding tube is placed, x-ray confirmation of placement is required before feeding is administered.	
___	___	___	10. If placement in stomach is not correct, untape tube, advance tube 5 cm, and repeat assessment in step 10.	
___	___	___	11. Secure tube by taping to bridge of patient's nose. Anchor tubing to patient's gown.	

PROCEDURE 32-4

Inserting a Nasogastric Tube *(Continued)*

Excellent	Satisfactory	Needs Practice		Comments
____	____	____	12. Clamp end of tubing or attach to suction, as ordered by healthcare provider.	
____	____	____	13. Wash hands, provide for patient's comfort, and remove equipment.	
____	____	____	14. Establish and document a plan for daily care of the nasogastric tube:	
____	____	____	a. Inspect nostril for irritation.	
____	____	____	b. Cleanse nostril frequently.	
____	____	____	c. Change adhesive as required to prevent skin irritation or pressure sores on nostril from the tube.	
____	____	____	d. Increase frequency of oral care because patients with nasogastric tubes often mouth breathe and may be NPO.	

Procedure Checklist for Fundamentals of Nursing: Human Health and Function, 7th edition

Name ______________________ Date ______________________

Unit ______________________ Position ______________________

Instructor/Evaluator: ______________________ Position ______________________

PROCEDURE 34-1

Pain Management: Patient-Controlled Analgesia

Excellent	Satisfactory	Needs Practice	**Goal:** Allow a patient to safely self-administer small preset doses of prescribed analgesic intravenously; with continuous infusion, allow a patient to receive a baseline continuous IV infusion of analgesic and also to safely self-administer small preset doses of prescribed analgesic as needed for increased pain.	**Comments**
___	___	___	1. Perform hand hygiene.	
___	___	___	2. Identify the patient.	
			Initiating PCA Therapy	
___	___	___	3. Close door or bed curtains and explain PCA to the patient:	
___	___	___	a. Explain to visitors/family that only the patient is to use the "pain button." Visitors/family may not push the pain button for the patient.	
___	___	___	b. Reinforce teaching throughout course of therapy.	
___	___	___	c. Document patient and family teaching.	
___	___	___	4. Check the prefilled syringe medication label against the medication order and the patient's identification. Some agencies require two nurses to double-check this step to ensure accuracy.	
___	___	___	5. Connect prefilled syringe to the PCA device tubing. Load syringe into PCA device.	
___	___	___	6. Prime PCA device tubing with the opioid medication. Program infusion dose and lockout interval according to the medication order.	
___	___	___	7. Lock PCA device and remove key.	
___	___	___	8. Clean port with antimicrobial swab. Connect the PCA device tubing to the patient's primary IV tubing. Activate PCA device by pressing the start button.	
___	___	___	9. Instruct patient to press button when experiencing pain. Reassure patient that lockout prevents possible overdose.	
___	___	___	10. Document administration of medication immediately, including date, time, dose, lockout interval, and any other observations of IV site and primary IV infusion.	

Excellent	Satisfactory	Needs Practice	PROCEDURE 34-1 **Pain Management: Patient-Controlled Analgesia** *(Continued)*	Comments
			Monitoring and Discontinuing PCA Therapy	
___	___	___	3. Close door or bed curtains and explain procedure to the patient.	
___	___	___	4. Check the IV site frequently for signs of infiltration or occlusion.	
___	___	___	5. If a patient is no longer capable of administering his or her medications, notify the physician so that another method of pain management can be used.	
___	___	___	6. If problems occur with the PCA, refer to the troubleshooting guide on the pump. The pain management nurse specialist, the pain team, or the IV team also can help with problems related to PCA.	
___	___	___	7. Using appropriate resources ensures safe administration. A physician's order is required for discontinuation of the PCA. Patients will often transition from IV medication to oral medication as they recover. An opioid transition order is required and will include directions that the registered nurse hold the PCA and deliver oral medications as prescribed. A "stop infusion" order is required once oral medications are evaluated for effectiveness and the infusion is discontinued.	
___	___	___	8. Discard all medication remaining in the opioid syringe in the presence of a second registered nurse. A second nurse witness is required for all wasted opioids. Record this information per individual hospital protocol.	
___	___	___	9. Record total medication dose (mg/mcg), milliliters (mL) infused, and milliliters (mL) left in the patient's record *every shift.*	
___	___	___	10. Document times of syringe changes on the MAR.	

Procedure Checklist for Fundamentals of Nursing: Human Health and Function, 7th edition

Name ______________________ Date ______________

Unit ______________________ Position ______________

Instructor/Evaluator: ______________________ Position ______________

PROCEDURE 34-2

Pain Management: Epidural Analgesia

Goal: Administer medications into the epidural or intrathecal space to control pain.

Excellent	Satisfactory	Needs Practice		Comments
___	___	___	1. Check physician order for current analgesia dose and complete six rights. The credentialed anesthesia provider who has placed the catheter has verified correct catheter placement and that the analgesia level of the patients is established and stabilized.	
___	___	___	2. Perform hand hygiene.	
___	___	___	3. Identify the patient using two separate identifiers.	
___	___	___	4. Close door or bed curtains and explain procedure to the patient.	
___	___	___	5. Insert tubing into medication bag; prime tubing and filter. Place tubing into color-coded pump with proper rate set to deliver ordered dose. Set limit to the amount of fluid in bag. Place epidural catheter label on tubing near pump.	
___	___	___	6. Cleanse connector of epidural catheter with Betadine swab. Wipe dry with sterile gauze.	
___	___	___	7. Recheck pump settings against physician's orders and turn on pump. Many agencies consider this a high-risk medication and require two nurses to double-check each other when the epidural infusion is started or changed.	
___	___	___	8. Follow medical orders for ongoing monitoring of pain level, vital signs, and sensorimotor function.	
___	___	___	9. Document any change in PCEA protocol adjustments along with the patient's response as they occur. At the end of shift, retrieve the total doses administered from epidural pump and clear the totals for the next shift. Record amount administered and amount remaining on the MAR.	

Procedure Checklist for Fundamentals of Nursing: Human Health and Function, 7th edition

Name ______________________ Date ______________________

Unit ______________________ Position ______________________

Instructor/Evaluator: ______________________ Position ______________________

PROCEDURE 35-1
Removing Contact Lenses

Goal: Remove contact lenses in the event that the patient is unable to do so.

Excellent	Satisfactory	Needs Practice	Step	Comments
___	___	___	1. Perform hand hygiene and identify the patient.	
___	___	___	2. Close door or bed curtains and explain the procedure to the patient, if possible.	
			Removing Hard Contact Lenses	
___	___	___	3. Position patient comfortably in a sitting position, if possible.	
___	___	___	4. Pull the patient's upper and lower lid apart and pull tautly toward the lateral side.	
___	___	___	5. Ask the patient to blink, and the lens should pop out into your hand.	
___	___	___	6. An alternative method for removing hard contact lenses is the use of a lens suction cup. This is particularly useful for a patient who cannot consciously assist with the removal.	
			Removing Soft Contact Lenses	
___	___	___	3. Position patient comfortably in a sitting position, if possible.	
___	___	___	4. Ask the patient to look upward. Pull down on the lower lid and place your index finger on the lower edge of the lens, moving it onto the white part of the eye	
___	___	___	5. Gently grasp lens between your thumb and index finger to release the suction of the lens. The lens will fold over and can easily be removed. Gently roll the lens, using normal saline as needed, to separate it and return it to its normal form.	
			Storing Lenses	
___	___	___	3. Rinse lenses thoroughly with recommended rinsing solution.	
___	___	___	4. Identify the left and right cups marked on the storage case.	
___	___	___	5. Place the first lens in its designated cup in the storage case before removing the second lens.	

Procedure Checklist for Fundamentals of Nursing: Human Health and Function, 7th edition

Name ______________________ Date ______________________

Unit ______________________ Position ______________________

Instructor/Evaluator: ______________________ Position ______________________

PROCEDURE 35-2

Assisting an Adult With Inserting a Hearing Aid

Excellent	Satisfactory	Needs Practice	**Goal:** Maintain hearing status; provide assistance with insertion.	**Comments**
___	___	___	1. Perform hand hygiene and identify the patient.	
___	___	___	2. Close door or bed curtains and explain the procedure to the patient, if possible.	
___	___	___	3. Check to be sure the battery is functional. Hold hearing aid in your hand and turn up the volume until you hear a "feedback" whistle. The feedback results from sound leaking around and back into the microphone and being amplified.	
___	___	___	4. Inspect the hearing aid to be sure that tubing and ear mold are intact and not cracked or broken. The opening in the ear mold should be free from cerumen.	
___	___	___	5. Clean hearing aid according to manufacturer's guidelines. Place in storage unit.	
___	___	___	6. Assess patient's ear for redness, irritation, drainage, and excessive cerumen. Moisten swab and clean ear as necessary.	
___	___	___	7. With the volume turned down, insert the ear mold into the ear canal, twisting slightly for a snug fit.	
___	___	___	8. Secure the battery behind the ear, if of that type. There are other styles of hearing aids that may fit in other ways.	
___	___	___	9. Turn the volume up slowly while speaking to the patient in a normal voice tone. Ask the patient to let you know when the sound level is comfortable.	